The
Rapid Recovery
Handbook

Elizabeth G. Motyka, MD,

Thomas M. Motyka, DO,

and Mark Nathaniel Mead, MSc

FOREWORD BY MEHMET C. OZ, MD

The Rapid Recovery Handbook

Your Complete Guide to
Faster Healing After Surgery

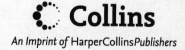 Collins

An Imprint of HarperCollinsPublishers

Disclaimer

This book will educate the reader about natural drugs, herbs, supplements, and complementary therapies. It is based on the personal experiences, research, and observations of the authors. This book is intended to be informational and by no means should be considered a substitute for advice from a licensed health professional, who should be consulted by the reader in matters relating to his or her health and particularly in respect to any symptoms that may require medical attention. While every effort has been made to ensure that selections of natural drugs, herbs, supplements, and other complementary therapies, and applicable dosages, are in accordance with current recommendations and practices, because of ongoing research and other factors, the reader is cautioned to check with a health professional about specific recommendations. In particular, readers who currently take prescription medications are cautioned to consult with a licensed health professional, ideally an integrative medicine practitioner with expertise in the use of neutriceuticals and botanicals, about specific recommendations for supplements and appropriate dosages. The authors and publisher expressly disclaim responsibility for any adverse effects arising from the use or application of the information contained in this book.

FIRST EDITION

Designed by Jaime Putorti

Library of Congress Cataloging-in-Publication Data has been requested.

ISBN-10: 0-06-074825-7
ISBN-13: 978-0-06-074825-8

06 07 08 09 10 WBC/RRD 10 9 8 7 6 5 4 3 2 1

To all those in need of healing.
In memory of William R. L. Mead.

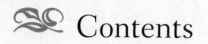 Contents

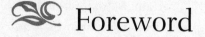 # Foreword

Sometimes difficult medical problems can only be "healed with steel." And yet when faced with imminent surgery, people often mistakenly believe that there's little they can do to influence the healing process and reduce the chances of a bad outcome. I disagree. How strongly you support your self-healing potential has a tremendous bearing on how well you recover from an operation. *The Rapid Recovery Handbook* speaks to the possibility of a happy marriage between the body's self-healing power and the curative power of surgery. It lays out a set of strategies that can accelerate the wound-healing process and arms you with the knowledge you need to help protect yourself and your loved ones from the potential setbacks that surgery can cause, all the while speeding up your return to good health.

It is heartening for me to see that various nutritional and physical care methods for expediting recovery after surgery are beginning to find their way into medical practice. Surgeons now understand that hypnosis, guided imagery, and other relaxation techniques can help patients relax before surgery and reduce the need for pain medications after surgery. Lessening the need for anti-inflammatory medication may in turn enable the natural healing process to proceed more rapidly.

The mind-body methods laid out in *The Rapid Recovery Handbook* have the power to make people feel more peaceful and in harmony as they head into an operation. These methods can also help you confront the myriad post-op challenges that can dramatically impact your life and the lives of family and friends. Emotional well-being, coupled with the promising nutritional and lifestyle interventions proposed by these authors, helps lay the biochemical groundwork for substantially improved healing.

Clearly, as these authors show, there's a great deal one can do to prevent unwanted outcomes and bring a quicker recovery. By providing so many wonderful tools to work with, this clearly written, well-organized book will empower you to take the right steps to bounce back physically after surgery. *The Rapid Recovery Handbook* is a must-read for anyone who finds themselves going under the knife.

Mehmet C. Oz, MD
Professor and Vice-chair of Surgery at NY Presbyterian-Columbia University Medical and Director of the Integrative Medicine Program

✑ Acknowledgments

We wish to thank Anne Cole, our editor at HarperCollins, for her brilliant editing, patience, wit, and attention to the myriad details of this book. We're also grateful to HarperCollins editor Gail Winston for her helpful feedback on the first draft, and to Barbara Motyka for her grammatical and stylistic suggestions on that initial draft. For additional support and encouragement along the way, we'd like to thank Sabine Mead, Keith and Penny Block, Suzanne Garman, Bernadette Bohmann, Kate Dunn, Lucie Branham, Vivian and Frank Gomba, Elena Schertz, Wendy Mann, John Breckenridge, Peter Guzzardi, Cynthia Runberg, Jonathan Fischer, Josh Alexander, John and Ginger Sall, Rivka From, Noriko Brantley, Bill Thomson, and all the librarians at the University of North Carolina's Health Sciences Library. Lastly, we wish to express our gratitude to all our patients who have offered valuable feedback about their personal healing experiences over the years.

The

Rapid Recovery
Handbook

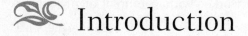 # Introduction

To help or at least to do no harm.
—HIPPOCRATIC OATH

One of the most dramatic experiences I remember from my medical student days was observing a woman having open abdominal surgery for advanced colon cancer. The precisely cut edges of the abdomen were being held open by the curved blades of a large steel instrument called a self-retaining retractor. In plain view were the liver, gallbladder, and intestines. A nearby monitor revealed a strong pulse and normal blood pressure. As I looked on, the surgeons skillfully wielded one instrument after another, and the entire procedure went off without a hitch. The surgical team then proceeded to close up the large gaping wound, successfully completing the operation.

Once the woman's abdomen had been carefully sown back together, it crossed my mind that everything was now up to the healing resources of the body. A biological task of monumental complexity lay ahead: the intricate healing of soft tissues, arteries, and skin, all of which would eventually result in the restoration of a normal, healthy, intact belly.

Every surgical scar tells a story that reflects this amazing healing potential. The story usually begins with an illness or some other event that creates the need for surgery, and then ends with the formation of mature scar tissue. It's what happens in between, and in particular how you can support your body in getting from point A to point B, that is the primary focus of this book. The untold story of every surgical scar is all the "little things" you do in terms of your nutrition, personal well-being, and other types of self-care to influence how well you heal from surgery. Our central premise in *The Rapid Recovery Handbook* is that your body's ability to heal itself simply should not be left to chance. It is entirely your choice to bolster this capacity and thereby speed up your recovery.

My personal interest in this area was sparked during college in the early 1980s. Throughout my undergrad years, I worked with a group of highly competent nurse midwives and learned about natural methods such as Lamaze breathing to help support women during labor and childbirth. I assisted midwives with births as well as in their teaching of childbirth classes. Prior to this experience, I had read Ina May Gaskin's classic work, *Spiritual Midwifery,* a book that introduced a whole generation of women to the concept of natural childbirth. Gaskin's book, along with my firsthand encounters with midwifery, helped plant the seeds for the kind of intimate connection I would one day cultivate with my patients.

As my senior year approached, I began to weigh my career options. Though I felt strongly aligned with midwifery's holistic philosophy and its proactive approach to healing, I was also wary of its limitations. In particular, I knew that I didn't want to feel dependent on others for the more specialized interventions that required medical expertise. I didn't want to find myself in the position of having to send a woman off to the operating room for a C-section or hysterectomy. Ultimately, it was my desire to be able to help people at every level of technical expertise that prompted me to apply to medical school. I went to med school with a clear awareness that I wanted to work in a holistic way, within an integrative medical setting.

During my first two years as a med student, I was strongly influenced by the thinking of Christiane Northrup, MD, a pioneer in the field of women's health. I felt inspired by the way she encouraged women to trust and fine-tune their own intuitive understanding of the body and its ever-changing patterns of health, a theme that became central to her book *Women's Bodies, Women's Wisdom.* Dr. Northrup constantly looked beyond the purely physical or somatic level to the mental, emotional, social, and spiritual context of health. If someone had a fibroid tumor, for example, she was interested in knowing why the fibroid might have grown in the first place, because such insights might help prevent it from recurring. Through her lectures and writings, Dr. Northrup opened my eyes to the burgeoning field of psychoneuroimmunology, the study of mind-body connections in relation to immunity and disease. I would later explore these connections with my own patients as they prepared for various procedures and wrestled with the causes and effects of disease.

While doing my residency at the University of North Carolina's School of Medicine, I felt glad to be in a place that had a recognized department of integrative medicine. The chairman of my department, Dr. William Droegemueller, was consistently upbeat about my interests, and when I began working as a physician, my first boss, Dr. Juan Granados, was similarly supportive. Even so, when I began to espouse this more holistic approach openly in the early 1990s, it was clear that I was working against the grain. My suggestions to patients were sometimes met with disapproval and bemusement on the part of the other physicians. As time went on, however, these same physicians began to refer patients to me, because it was clear that patients were seeking and benefiting from an integrative approach to health care.

Among the more lasting insights I gleaned from my surgical training—an insight that would profoundly inform my evolution as a practitioner of integrative medicine—was the pivotal role of the body's *stress response* in the aftermath of surgery. The stress response encompasses an array of hormonal and metabolic changes that take place in the body following physical trauma or injury, and many of these same changes tend to complicate the healing process while adding to the various problems that go along with surgery.

With experience, every surgeon learns to cultivate a healthy respect for the stress response. The standard approach is to rely on medications to blunt the response; however, this strategy can have negative effects and actually makes the person less resilient in the aftermath of surgery. My inclination is to depend more on natural methods like herbal therapy, acupuncture, and relaxation techniques—techniques that can dramatically decrease the need for medications while fortifying the body's self-healing system.

My personal interest in the stress response led me to study the work of Dr. Herbert Benson, founding president of Harvard's Mind/Body Medical Institute, and Dr. Jon Kabat-Zinn, who developed the now-famous Stress Reduction Program at the University of Massachusetts. These studies led me to incorporate hypnosis and various relaxation exercises to help my patients prepare for minor surgeries. For example, I encouraged patients to visualize a beautiful scene to help the body relax more deeply before the start of an operation. (I recall several occasions during which nurses on my staff would almost doze off while I read a relaxation script to a patient—clearly, they were in need of stress reduction as well!) Once I saw that patients were much less tense and experienced less pain during minor procedures, I started recommending these techniques for major surgeries as well. The central tenet of these strategies is that we support the body in doing its job rather than muddling the healing process by relying too much on medications.

Good nutrition, of course, simply makes sense from a surgical standpoint. Many people looking for a holistic or integrative approach are also looking for ways to improve their nutrition. When they ask their medical team about this aspect, most are told that they simply need to follow a "healthy diet" or a "well-balanced eating plan." They are told that supplements are unnecessary since the essential nutrients can be obtained from a wide array of foods. Unfortunately, most of the people handing out this simplistic advice have never really had much nutrition training. The truth is that supplements are almost always helpful because of the fact that surgery imposes considerable nutritional stresses on the body. The body goes into a high-intensity metabolic state immediately after surgery, which depletes the very nutrients it needs to heal efficiently. Supplementation can help bolster the healing process even when the diet is considered "well balanced."

My husband, Tom, an osteopathic physician, has strongly influenced my understanding of the power of nutrition. When I first met Tom, he already had studied the nutrition teachings of Drs. Wally Schmidt, Paavo Airola, Michael Murray, Leo Galland, and Jeff Bland. He also had formal studies of nutrition through his osteopathic training and through his graduate studies at the University of North Carolina's School of Public Health. Over the past decade, Tom and I have sought ways to improve the nutrition of patients who were facing, or had undergone, surgery. Our initial motivation for doing this was simple. When we began questioning patients about their health habits before and after an operation, it quickly became clear to us that the ones who had a healthy diet and took multivitamins recovered much more smoothly. This only reinforced our conviction that nutrition and other natural healing methods were essential to help patients get better.

It wasn't long before we had begun to advise all our surgical patients to follow a balanced diet and take a multivitamin supplement, to quit smoking and drinking, and to use relaxation tapes before the operation. In addition, we recommended safe and effective natural therapies that would help them feel and function better on a daily basis.

A few years ago, I left the university system and started a private practice with Tom. At the university, many of my surgical patients had come from less-fortunate circumstances such as migrant worker families, the prison system, and other underserved populations. In our private practice, by contrast, most patients were better educated and already were doing many things conducive to good health. Many were following high-fiber, vegetable-rich diets, taking nutritional supplements, exercising, and taking steps to reduce their stress level. Once again, patients in this healthier context appeared to be faring better in the wake of surgery—certainly better than the majority of patients I had cared for at the teaching hospital. They had fewer wound infections and faster wound healing in general. This awareness prompted Tom and me to look even deeper into some of the ways that natural healing methods could be fine-tuned to improve healing in the postoperative period. In addition to nutritional suggestions, we advised patients to engage in acupuncture, massage, and other body-centered therapies. The benefits we have seen from this integrative medicine approach continue to surprise and impress us to this day.

In mid-October 2001, Mark Mead, a well-known health writer and nutrition research consultant in our community, was meeting with Tom before having knee surgery. The operation would involve a complete reconstruction of his anterior cruciate ligament, or ACL, and Mark wanted Tom's opinion on what his chances were for a speedy recovery. As an osteopathic physician, Tom had worked with many patients recovering from ACL reconstruction and other orthopedic surgeries. He had a special connection with Mark, as the two had attended the University of North Carolina's School of Public Health together and played on the same basketball team in the Chapel Hill recreation league. Now Mark was coming to Tom after having injured his knee playing basketball.

When Mark came limping into our clinic on that cool and breezy October day, Tom gave him a comprehensive evaluation, and then Mark popped the question: "So what would you do if you were in my shoes and wanted to get back on the basketball court as soon as possible?" Tom gave his opinion on the value of glucosamine and other nutritional aides for improving surgical healing of the joint area. Together they came up with a combination of nutritional and body-centered strategies that would complement the physical therapy routine recommended by Mark's surgeon, Dr. William Garrett, who is presently a professor of surgery at Duke University and director of the American Board of Orthopaedic Surgery.

Dr. Garrett had told Mark after the surgery that he likely would be in considerable pain and discomfort for several days to a week after the operation. It would be several months, the surgeon predicted, before the swelling had disappeared, and at least 10 months before he could resume a regular exercise routine. Dr. Garrett cautioned Mark that he probably would never recover his former range of motion and advised him to start thinking of other sports he could play besides basketball, his favorite form of exercise. Mark says that he went home that day determined more than ever to maintain his nutrition-based rapid repair program.

I should point out that Mark already had maintained a wholesome fiber- and micronutrient-rich diet before coming to our clinic, and his in-depth studies of nutrition had led him to explore a variety of supplement options to support tissue repair. These options included, among other things, a high-quality omega-3 fatty acid supplement, the Power Healing Drink (which we introduce in chapter 4), and a potent "joint support formula" that contained high concentrations of glucosamine, buffered vitamin C, and MSM (methylsulfonylmethane), an organic source of sulfur utilized by the body in the formation of connective tissue. To this, Tom added bromelain, turmeric, and boswellia, anti-inflammatory herbals that had shown promise in a number of studies. Magnetic therapy was also part of Mark's regimen, as he had come across several clinical trials showing that small magnets, placed at specific locations in proximity to an inflamed joint, reduced pain and swelling. In addition, for relaxation and pleasure, Mark regularly practiced a gentle moving meditation sequence that he had developed after years of studying the ancient martial art known as tai chi.

Within a few weeks of the operation, all the swelling around his knee had dissipated. Mark's physical therapists were astonished when they observed that he could bend his knee beyond 45 degrees at 3 months. They told Mark to stay with the nutrition and herbal program, because he was on the same recovery line as the eighteen-year-old college athletes they were seeing who had undergone the same surgery. For Mark, who was in his early forties, this kind of feedback confirmed that what he was doing was right on track.

Four months later, Mark was back to playing full-court basketball just as well as he'd ever played. The experience confirmed for him the power of nutritional and herbal support in the healing process. As Mark told us during one follow-up visit, there were times when he would look down at his knee and ask himself whether the surgeon had slipped him a new leg during the operation. The speedy repair had enabled him to reclaim most of the strength, stability, flexibility, and range of motion in the once injured leg. He felt balanced and energized after each workout.

When Mark returned for his final follow-up visit to our office, the three of us discussed how many patients having surgery could benefit from such an accelerated repair program. I told Mark that his suggestion for *The Rapid Recovery Handbook* was just what I was looking for as a guide for patients planning elective surgery. I told him how Tom and I had been continually impressed with the ease and rapidity of recovery that came with using specific superfoods, supplements, and other self-healing tools around the time of surgery, and in the months after. The three of us decided then and there to coauthor *The Rapid Recovery Handbook*.

The book you have in your hands is designed to give you tools and strategies to enhance your innate wound-healing potential and to increase your chances of a speedy recovery after surgery. We feel confident that the information will be of great value to anyone facing an imminent surgery as well as those who have recently had surgery and want to get back to normal functioning as soon as possible. We've organized each of the chapters to allow you to explore those strategies that are most relevant to your particular situation—whether you're about to have an operation or have recently had surgery—in order to ensure the most successful recovery and long-term health.

Some readers will be able to take advantage of *all* our tips—in particular, those who face an elective surgery and still have plenty of time beforehand. The first three chapters explain how the body heals, the nutritional basics for healing, and the rationale for our rapid recovery program. Chapters 4 and 5 reveal a program for before and during surgery. If your operation is far more imminent—say, within a few days—you may want to read chapters 4 and 5 first. Even for people who have been through surgery, the diet and mind-body suggestions in chapters 4 and 5, respectively, will be helpful. If the operation already has been performed, then you may want to start with chapter 6 and read the postoperative program and remaining chapters first. Wherever you are in the healing process, this program can help ease and expedite your recovery.

Our own clinical experience continues to validate the immense potential of optimizing your nutrition, herbal support, and overall self-care around the time of surgery and in the weeks and months that follow. A number of the strategies we describe in this book will support your overall functioning and vitality long after the operation. Having witnessed the success of so many patients who have followed our advice, we feel confident that the guidance we provide here will be invaluable for speeding up your recovery.

—Elizabeth Motyka, MD

1

At the Cutting Edge
of Surgical Care

. . . and not until the wound heals
and the scar disappears,
do we begin to discover where we are,
and that nature is
one and continuous everywhere.

—Henry David Thoreau

Why do some people seem to recover so much faster than others who have the same surgery under the same circumstances? How much does your own state of health influence the healing process postsurgery, and what can you do to make sure that your recovery unfolds as smoothly and rapidly as possible?

Some of what affects how tissues heal has to do with the surgery itself—specifically, the type of procedure, the surgical technique, the operating room environment, and most of all your surgeon's level of expertise. Those factors largely depend on your surgical team, though, as we'll see in chapter 5, you can request various environmental conditions to be in place during your operation. But there's much more to it than that. A number of practical steps can be taken before, during, and after the procedure to increase your self-healing ability. Among the starting points are some simple lifestyle choices, including the kinds of foods you eat and the dietary supplements you use before and after the operation.

All too often, the importance of nutrition has received short shrift in mainstream medical practice, though there are signs of change on the horizon. In a report titled "Fit for Surgery," published in the December 2004 issue of *Surgeon,* experts from six European countries and the United States addressed the issue of how best to prepare patients for surgery. Malnutrition was placed at the top of the list of factors that can impede recovery after surgery. "Malnutrition is common among hospitalized patients and in the community, while patients' nutritional status often declines during hospital stay," the report stated. "Both malnutrition and weight loss are associated with alterations in cellular physiology and organ function, which are of importance for the surgical patient. Preoperative malnutrition compromises surgical outcome while preoperative weight loss can lead to increased postoperative morbidity and mortality." The report went on to note that nutritional assessments are rarely done on people facing surgery, despite the fact that malnutrition is common among hospitalized patients. Moreover, the authors noted: "In order to ensure that patients undergoing elective procedures are 'fit for surgery,' all members of the multidisciplinary team should understand that adequate nutrition contributes to a successful surgical outcome."[1]

Of course, making sure that you have sufficient or *adequate* nutrition to handle the rigors of surgery is key. In *The Rapid Recovery Handbook,* however, we're more interested in *optimum* nutrition than in *adequate* nutrition. We will teach you about the best possible combinations of foods, nutrients, and nutriceuticals (including herbal supplements), for maximizing your healing potential. To reinforce and enhance the impact of this nutrition, we'll explore mind-body techniques, therapeutic exercise, physical manipulation, energy medicine, and other easily accessible, noninvasive tools that have been shown to support optimal wound repair. These considerations, as you will learn, can be of tremendous benefit. They will enable you to go through surgery with greater ease and comfort, and to recover as fast as is humanly possible after your operation.

❧ The Many Flavors and Challenges of Surgery

Surgery is the medical specialty that treats diseases or injuries through operations or what physicians refer to as "procedures." Many surgeries are aimed at removing or repairing a part of the body, or at establishing whether a disease is present. Surgery can also involve transplantation of organs, tissues, or cells from one site to another within the same individual, or from one patient to another of the same species or even of different species. Other surgeries focus on problems that develop in the bones, joints, and ligaments of the human body. Still others are performed in order to repair or restore body parts to look normal, or to change a body part to look better. And the list goes on.

Many surgeries are either lifesaving or at least potentially lifesaving procedures. Consider, for example, the removal of a large tumor that is impinging on a vital organ. Curative surgery is regarded as the primary treatment for most cancers. Today, more-conservative (less-invasive) surgeries are aimed at removing tumors while preserving as much normal tissue and function as possible. These sophisticated procedures offer the greatest chance for cure for common cancers like those of the breast, prostate, and colon—as long as the cancer has not yet spread to other parts of the body.

Or consider the miracle of coronary bypass, which involves using a piece of vein or artery to bypass a blockage in a coronary artery in order to prevent heart attacks or to relieve chest pain due to reduced blood flow to heart muscles. For quite some time now, cardiovascular disease has been the leading cause of death in the United States, and today more than 60 percent of cardiovascular-related deaths are linked with coronary artery disease. With the increasing size of the middle-aged and elderly population, more bypass operations will need to be performed on people confronting this disease.

Other examples of major surgery include brain surgery, hysterectomy, mastectomy, joint reconstruction, joint replacement, organ transplants, or bone marrow transplants. Regardless of which type you're facing, it usually promises to be a significant event that can severely tax your body's healing resources. Substantial risks may be involved, and our clinical experience has shown us over and over again that the surgically treated body can greatly benefit from targeted support to help minimize these risks. Major surgery also tends to result in extensive tissue loss as well as a major restructuring of tissue. Your body must be sufficiently healthy to mount an efficient healing response to such damage.

A number of setbacks or complications can occur after major surgery or with a series of operations—setbacks like heart problems and postoperative depression. Other common problems include pain, nausea, decreased bowel and bladder function, lack of mobility, or immune dysfunction. These types of problems, when they come up, can become worse during your hospitalization or during your rehab at home. People in these situations need advice on how to guard against these health glitches, function well during the recovery phase, and get back to normal as quickly as possible.

Fortunately, many of the tactics that help you prevent these surgery-related setbacks in the first place dovetail nicely with those that make for better healing after surgery. For example good nutrition not only promotes healing, it can help prevent infection. Also, as you'll learn in chapter 6, the stressful effects of surgery may hinder healing *and* set the stage for various setbacks to occur with greater force and frequency. Whether you're about to undergo surgery or recently had it, the strategies we describe for dealing with these stressful effects can give you just the advantage you need to get back to a place of stability, balance, and optimal functioning in your life.

Be Proactive About Your Surgery

With recent medical advances, more and more people are opting for elective surgery, meaning that you essentially get to choose when and where to have the surgery, and whether you even want the surgery in the first place. About 8 out of every 10 surgeries are elective. For this reason, it's increasingly important to pay attention to your repair and recovery period as pressures on nursing and hospital resources continue to mount. With burgeoning hospital bureaucracies, federal regulations, bloated insurance companies, and attempts to micromanage doctors leading to exorbitant medical costs, cost cutting has become the order of the day. More than ever before, patients are being discharged sooner after major surgery, hoisting a greater responsibility for a complete recovery on the patient.

Against this challenging backdrop, you cannot afford to be too complacent about your body's ability to mount the fastest possible recovery from surgery. In the chapters that follow, we will offer you some scientifically based suggestions for specific nutrient combinations, mind-body techniques, and other easily accessible, noninvasive tools to optimize your healing potential. This program will not only enable you to go through surgery with greater ease and comfort, but also to recover faster after your operation.

Understand Your Self-Healing Repertoire

Ordinarily, the task of supporting your recovery after surgery is assigned to a physical therapist or to the nursing staff, or both. After the operation, you may be told how to use medications and ice. You may be shown how to breathe deeply and change positions in bed. You will be advised to carry out certain exercises as soon as possible after the operation. These postoperative activities can and do help the body heal by increasing blood circulation and thus the flow of oxygen, reducing muscle discomfort, and preventing complications in vital organ systems. But they represent only one piece of the wound-healing puzzle. *The Rapid Recovery Handbook* lays out this puzzle as an integrated whole, as a system for repair and healing that can be used in conjunction with the more conventional forms of support mentioned above.

Throughout this book, we highlight dietary and lifestyle habits that can bolster your self-healing capacities, and alert you to habits can have a negative impact. This is the most basic step in any healing program. We also explain why it's just as important to remove those "antihealing" factors from your diet and lifestyle as it is to incorporate the ones that have healing effects.

We've arranged the self-healing tools you will need to help your body recover from surgery into four basic groups: (1) nutritional and botanical strategies; (2) lifestyle changes; (3) body-centered care; and (4) mind-body strategies. You can think of these tools simply in the following way. Nutrition and botanicals give the body what it needs to heal, the raw materials you often need more of after surgery. Exercise and body-centered therapy help the body get what it needs—oxygen, vitamins, and other nutrients—while supporting immunity, detoxification, and neuromuscular functioning, thereby helping in the wound-healing process in more subtle ways. Lifestyle habits and mind-body strategies help combat day-to-day conditions that get in the way of healing. All four work together in an intimate collaboration to make sure your healing phase is as smooth and effective as possible.

Of course, most likely your physician will prescribe certain drugs to assist with pain and inflammation. Even so, the self-healing tools we recommend can be useful, reducing your need for costly medications and the risk of becoming dependent on these pharmaceuticals. By making yourself less dependent on inflammatory drugs, you not only cut costs but also speed up your own healing process.

❧ How to Use This Handbook

This book is organized according to the three phases of surgery. The first phase is the *preoperative period,* in which you prepare your body for the dramatic effects of major surgery and up your chances of responding well to the event. Emergency surgeries will generally preclude any form of preparation. For people facing elective surgery, however, the preparation can be substantial, in most cases at least several weeks, if not several months. If the surgery is relatively minor, such as a vasectomy, your efforts during the preoperative period will generally be less important. Nonetheless, there are factors in your nutrition, physical care, and mind-body awareness that can virtually make *any* surgery and its aftermath a more positive experience.

The second phase, called the *intraoperative period,* includes the actual operation as well as a brief period of mind-body preparation just before the operation. Among the mind-body techniques you may consider during this phase are meditation, self-hypnosis, and guided imagery. Some of these techniques may be as short as five minutes. Environmental conditions, too, are a good thing to think about: ensuring that you have plenty of oxygen, a warm temperature in the operating room, and soothing music during the operation. Your surgeon may set up these conditions before the operation, though most likely you will have to request them. These and other considerations are relevant if you're receiving full anesthesia during the operation. For people facing only local or regional anesthesia, mind-body practices may be helpful during the actual surgery.

The third and final phase is the *postoperative period,* or what you do after the operation. Logically, most of *The Rapid Recovery Handbook* focuses on this period. Here is where practical efforts to expedite tissue repair and recovery have their greatest impact. Most of the nutritional strategies we recommend relate to the post-op period, as do physical therapy (or other body-centered therapies) and stress reduction techniques. The good news is that even if you're reading this book soon after your operation, there's still much you can do to bolster your body's internal repair resources and help you reenter your life in tip-top condition as quickly as possible.

Dealing with Scientific Evidence

You can use this book in two ways: (1) to identify the foods, supplements, and therapies you think might expedite your recovery; and (2) to convince health care professionals you're working with to give at least some of these approaches a try. Of course, you will first need to be able to answer this fundamental question: How do I know whether a particular food, supplement, or therapy has some value as a tool for speeding up my recovery from surgery?

The answer is more complicated than you might expect. Many of the natural approaches have scientific merit based only on clinical observations on a case-by-case basis. This is known as anecdotal evidence, and it is often much maligned by proponents of mainstream medicine, even though anecdotal observations are frequently harbingers of major medical breakthroughs.

Other natural approaches have scientific merit based on animal studies, cell culture studies, or other forms of laboratory research. And yet there isn't much clinical trial research to back up the creation of standard guidelines for physicians. Randomized, double-blind, placebo-controlled clinical trials are considered to be the gold standard of scientific research. Such studies are particularly useful because they greatly minimize sources of bias that can alter the outcome and therefore distort the true effect. Clinical trial evidence can be found in abundance for many drug-related treatments, and for good reason: these drugs and invasive procedures can have serious side effects if used improperly, and the majority of cases (over-the-counter medications excepted) will require your physician to prescribe or otherwise intervene.

When it comes to natural options such as foods, nutrients, or herbs, however, there is often a lack of such high-level evidence. The main reason for this is that most of these agents or interventions are not patentable and therefore will not attract the kind of research funding that's required for the testing of pharmaceuticals. Even where clinical trial evidence does exist, it may not be reliable because insufficient dosage levels of nutrients or botanicals may have been used. Against this backdrop, it may be tempting to dismiss the use of nutrients or botanicals. Nonetheless, as long as questions of safety have been resolved, we believe there are often strong grounds for incorporating these natural options into your self-care plan. Our goal is not to provide a comprehensive review of all the studies that have been done on the use of natural agents and therapies as a way to speed healing after surgery. Some of the strategies and agents have more scientific support than others, and we've elected to elaborate on research in particular areas to back up certain points or to highlight the power of a specific perspective. For the areas that are more scientifically questionable, we will offer the appropriate caveats and suggestions for safe use. We have made every effort to be rigorous about the studies we've included and our interpretations of them.

Before closing, we'd like to a make a brief statement about how the general public perceives and understands science. This perception is heavily colored by the simplistic manner in which the media shares scientific reports with the public today. New health studies are released daily to the media, but what writers, editors, and publishers are usually looking for is the most sensational or startling angle on a particular topic. The media reporter's imperative, moreover, is to boil down these findings into simple sound bites that inadvertently mislead the public or paint a lopsided picture of the evidence to date.

As an example, we recently heard on the news that the popular antiarthritis supplement, a combination of glucosamine and chondroitin, was no better than placebo "dummy pills" at relieving arthritis pain in a large clinical trial published in the February 2006 issue of the *New England Journal of Medicine*. This was indeed the general finding for the whole group—that is, for all the study participants put together. What the media failed to mention, however, was that those patients with *moderate-to-severe* pain who took glucosamine with chondroitin did show a *statistically significant 25 percent reduction* in pain compared to the placebo group. Media reports also overlooked the fact that well over a dozen randomized controlled trials had already demonstrated the painkilling benefits of this supplement in the context of osteoarthritis. (Similarly, the media reported in 2005 that the common herb echinacea was ineffective against the common cold, based on a single study, and yet at least 14 randomized clinical trials had previously shown a beneficial impact on colds and other upper respiratory infections. Shortly afterward, another herb, Saint-John's-wort, was said to have failed against depression, despite the fact that dozens of clinical trials had demonstrated its antidepressant power.)

There are numerous other examples of recent media reports that have triggered a great deal of confusion in the world of nutrition and nutriceuticals. One of these focused on the famous Women's Health Initiative (WHI) study, which has tracked nearly 161,000 women for 15 years, comparing those on a regular diet to those on a low-fat diet. Scientists met for several days to try to report the findings of this huge and costly trial. Meanwhile, as usual, newspapers nationwide trumpeted the study's most general findings—namely, that dietary fat did not help prevent cancer and heart disease, and that calcium had no bearing on osteoporosis. Once again, though, closer scrutiny of the original findings revealed that fat and calcium intakes did make a significant difference for certain groups within the study: women with the largest decrease in fat intake had a 21 percent reduction in breast cancer: those who ate the least saturated fat and hydrogenated fat showed a 15 percent reduction in heart disease; and women over sixty who took their calcium supplements had a nearly 30 percent reduction in hip fractures. The WHI study therefore had many valuable lessons that were obscured by media reports. By no means did it show that a low-fat diet and calcium supplementation were of no value!

Our point here is that you have to read past the headlines to get the big picture. When reporters try to simplify findings, they invariably ignore the more valuable implications of a study, and the end result is "sound bite science." Also remember that science itself is often a murky process. No single study can offer definitive proof to discount a particular hypothesis. And studies of whole populations may not necessarily be relevant to you, the individual. Recommendations for populations can be very different from individual recommendations, which is why a clinically tailored approach, one guided primarily by your own physician's judgment and experience, is so vitally important.

Your ability to heal, a direct reflection of your body's innate wisdom, may be more powerful than you think. We believe the practical guidance contained in this book will help you unlock the secrets to that deeper wisdom. This information will help you immensely around the time of surgery and for many months after an operation. May your journey toward rapid repair and recovery be filled with the deeper pleasures of enduring health and vitality. So now that you've been introduced to our thinking and to the basic plan for using *The Rapid Repair Handbook,* let's get started!

2

The Art and Science
of Wound Healing

Surgeons must be careful
When they take the knife
Underneath their fine incisions
Stirs the Culprit—Life!

—EMILY DICKINSON

At age forty-one, Elena B. had come to me in search of holistic approaches to treat her heavy menstrual cycles. She had gotten some relief from using natural progesterone cream and acupuncture, but it was short-lived. To further reduce her circulating estrogen levels, we then tried various dietary changes—avoiding high-fat, hormone-laden animal products and eating more vegetables and fruits, whole grains, and fish—and supplemented with a multivitamin specifically formulated for women. The flow lessened a bit, but the pain and discomfort continued and began to interfere with her job as a physical therapist. On some days the flow was so intense that she felt she couldn't even leave the house. This left her homebound for several days each month. I suggested oral contraceptives, which are often effective in such situations, but Elena could not tolerate these drugs—they triggered migraine headaches.

By age forty-three, Elena felt that she had exhausted the medical alter-

natives. After getting a second opinion and consulting with me once more to carefully weigh her options, she opted for a solution that had a well-documented success rate: surgery. Now Elena came to me with a new set of questions. She wanted to know how best to prepare her body, mind, and spirit for the surgery. Having been interested in natural medicine for many years, she initiated her own search on the Internet, visiting multiple Web sites and chat rooms for several weeks. On weekends, she browsed her local bookstores to glean information on nutrition, mind-body methods, and botanical aids to healing. As a gynecologic surgeon, I had performed thousands of different surgeries, and had some very definite ideas of what had worked well for my patients over the years. Elena and I met several times to discuss these strategies as well as those that she had learned about in her own information search.

After reviewing her options and the various risks and benefits, Elena decided to go ahead with surgery to address the excessively long periods and heavy bleeding. She decided to have endometrial ablation, a procedure that destroys a thin layer of the lining of the uterus. The procedure is done in the operating room under either IV sedation or general anesthesia, but is far less invasive and much less debilitating than hysterectomy, and the reproductive organs are spared. A number of my patients have responded very well to endometrial ablation, which usually stops all menstrual flow in about 50 percent of patients and decreases flow to light bleeding or spotting afterward in another 30 percent. The procedure can involve a variety of electric-surgical techniques as well cryogenic surgery (using liquid nitrogen) and a microwave electrical method. Those women who don't respond to the procedure will usually go on to have a hysterectomy.

In the course of helping Elena decide between a hysterectomy and endometrial ablation, she and I had discussed the typical course of recovery and repair. This gave me the opportunity to explain the stages of wound healing and how nutrition, relaxation, bodywork, and lifestyle choices could be timed to accelerate her return to a normal, healthy life.

Like many surgical patients who come to me for integrative care, Elena was highly motivated to have a rapid recovery. After discussing her diet and current lifestyle, we decided to schedule the operation in six weeks so she could optimize her preoperative nutrition and mind-body preparation. She agreed to modify her diet in the interim, beginning with the removal of all refined carb foods—namely, pastries, cakes, and other white flour products. Her biggest challenge was giving up butter and french fries. I suggested that she substitute a no-trans-fat spread like Earth Balance for butter and try baked skin-on fries with olive oil. She began consuming more whey protein and phytonutrients with the help of our Power Healing Drink (see recipe, page 73) in the morning. She supplemented with a multivitamin, as well as additional vitamin C and some omega-3 fatty acids. As she was having a minor procedure, these changes were all that we decided she needed to make. She was very motivated to recovery quickly and did not find it too difficult to make these changes. We fortunately have three superb organic health food stores in our area, so she had no trouble obtaining the foods and supplements I suggested.

Over the weeks leading up to the surgery, Elena practiced using relaxation techniques to help decrease the stressful impact of the surgery on her body. She was already doing a yoga class once a week and added listening and breathing with a relaxation tape at bedtime to her routine. The afternoon of her surgery, she looked relaxed and in control as we wheeled her into the operating room. She listened to her music and relaxation script on her iPOD headphones, requiring only a light sedation for anesthetic. A few hours after the procedure, she returned home to continue her program. She was ecstatic about the 95 percent reduction in bleeding during her cycle, and felt healthy and energized to step back into her practice and family life. Within two weeks she was back to working full-time and was able to go bike riding with her husband and two kids during her light periods. No more staying at home in bed!

—EGM

The human body is a self-healing miracle. Over the course of evolution, it has developed an astounding capacity for replacing old and damaged tissue—and remaining vital in the process. These restorative processes are ongoing. For instance, you create a new stomach lining every 5 days. The liver, your body's biochemical mastermind, completes a new cycle of regeneration every 6 weeks. You don a new skin about once a month, while your bones and red blood cells reconstitute themselves about every 3 months. So it is that the pulsation of life calls on us to renew our bodies constantly, right down to the cells and molecules that comprise our flesh and blood.

Underlying this powerful capacity for ongoing renewal is a cellular intelligence that enables us to respond in a highly constructive way to physical injury or wounds of one form or another. So efficient is the wound-healing process in most cases that you're unlikely to pay much attention to minor cuts or scratches. Such superficial wounds are passed off as a temporary irritation, since you know, at least intuitively, that your body has the resources to mend within a few days. Major gashes, throbbing sores, or festering wounds will, of course, prompt some first-aid action, at the very least cleaning, dressing, and bandaging the wound. Nonetheless, as long as your health is reasonably good, there is an abiding faith that even these more onerous wounds will disappear in time. Major wounds may take weeks or even months to heal, but in the end the result is the same: tissues mend, and only a scar—if that—remains to remind us of the original event.

Surgery itself—the primary focus of this book—involves the deliberate creation of a wound, usually by making a very careful incision. The more radical forms of surgery result in more serious wounds and thus require longer and more labor-intensive recoveries. With any type of surgery, however, the practical key to a smooth and speedy recovery lies in your body's self-healing capacities—your internal resources for optimal tissue repair.

While many health books for the general public have addressed recovery from surgery and other medical situations, the issue of how to support tissue repair—the wound-healing process—has been largely overlooked. *Repair* refers to an intricate process by which the healing of damaged tissue takes place at the molecular and cellular levels. The body's repair mechanisms are triggered in response to any form of injury. This is a systemic process, meaning that it requires the integration of several bodily systems—namely, the circulatory, immune, hemostatic (blood regulating), hormonal, and nervous systems—and the connective tissues found throughout the body. Our clinical experience indicates that an integrative approach is the best way to fully support each of these systems, thereby ensuring that tissue repair will occur as smoothly and efficiently as possible.

The term *recovery*, in contrast with *repair*, refers to the experience of getting back to a normal level of functioning and overall performance. Obviously, recovery speed will depend, in large part, on how quickly and completely your body can repair the wound after the operation. The macrocosm called recovery depends heavily upon the microcosm called repair. While a return to normal functioning often *will* occur in time, any effort to accelerate repair will make recovery more efficient, more pleasant, and ultimately more satisfying in the long run.

As physicians and researchers with expertise in integrative medicine, we've further expanded the definition of recovery. Again, our goal is to help you realize or reclaim an *optimal* level of functioning—a degree of peak performance that makes your daily life more fulfilling, productive, and enjoyable. Surgery should improve function, not just remove disease. To attain peak performance, your regenerative capacities need to be taken to the highest level possible. This calls for supporting your body's self-healing mechanisms and bolstering overall health in a logical, scientifically grounded manner.

✒ Aging and Metabolic Individuality: Why Some of Us Recover Faster

The majority of surgeries are uneventful in terms of recovery. Nevertheless, the fact remains that some people heal much more quickly and smoothly than others. Any two people undergoing the same operation can have radically different experiences of recovery.

In recent years, we've come a long way toward understanding the basis for these different outcomes. Each of us has a unique ability to repair tissue and tolerate the physical assaults of surgery. Much of this ability is determined by what might be called *biological age*. When people ask how old someone is, they are usually referring to chronological age, a number determined, quite simply, by how many times each of us has traveled around the sun. Biological age is a subtler concept. It's a measure of the biological integrity of our cells and tissues. This, in turn, translates into our overall health and vitality. With biological age, it's possible to be fifty years old yet have the strength and flexibility of a forty-year-old, or perhaps someone much younger.

The aging process has a pivotal place in the individualized nature of recovery. When we're young, our tissues heal very quickly. When you were a child playing outdoors during the summer, you may have skinned your knees on a number of occasions. These superficial wounds typically mended in a matter of days—unless, of course, you skinned your knee in the same place in the interim.

As we age, though, our wound-healing response becomes more sluggish. Grandparents undergoing an appendectomy, bypass operation, or orthopedic surgery will typically take three to four times longer to heal compared to their teenage grandchildren. This is just the natural order of things: aging means a slowing down of one's regenerative capacity.

In some cases, the body's self-healing resources may be so compromised by the effects of advanced age that major surgery becomes extremely risky, if not prohibitive. The long-range solution, of course, is to take better care of those internal resources that enable wound healing to take place as we grow older—via good nutrition, regular exercise, stress management, and a nontoxic and noninflammatory lifestyle.

One of the ways we can get an even better handle on our biological age is by using antioxidant supplements as well as natural agents that support how our glands function, in particular the pituitary and pineal glands. It is known, for example, that the pituitary gland produces smaller amounts of growth hormone as we grow older. But nutritional supplements, as well as good sleep and stress management, can greatly improve your pituitary gland's production of growth hormone and the various other growth factors it triggers.[1] These growth factors collectively play a vital role in the process of wound healing.

On Blaming the Gene Pool

Genetics, like the aging process, has an integral role in the wound healing biodrama. Our genes provide the basic blueprint for the manufacture of enzymes, hormones, and other substances our bodies need when dealing with the duress of surgery. Some bodies are genetically more resistant to the damaging effects of surgery, while others are more vulnerable. In particular, some bodies are genetically predisposed to chronic inflammation, which can lead to a higher level of discomfort after the surgery, as well as more frequent complications and a slower recovery overall.

We have little direct control over our genetic makeup: quite literally, what we inherit is what we get. But our health at any given moment is much more than a matter of genetic destiny. Genes do not exist and function in isolation; they constantly interact with the body's own chemistry. The biochemistry we create through a health-promoting diet and lifestyle is the same biochemistry that supports the healthy expression of our genes. It is the same biochemistry that supports our genes' ability to bolster immunity, keep inflammation under control, improve tolerance to pain, and accelerate wound healing.

✌ Your First Priority: Remove Healing Impediments

Whether you've been told you need surgery or you're considering an elective procedure, there are many steps you can take to bolster your body's repair mechanisms. Although we cannot change our age and genetics there are many outside factors that can be controlled. By getting rid of what prevents good wound healing, you're in a much better place to speed up the process.

Overusing medications. The first factor to look at is whether you're taking too much medication or the wrong ones. Potent anti-inflammatory drugs can impede tissue repair by suppressing your body's inflammatory response, which is integral to the wound-healing process.* For this reason, chronic, high-dose use of ibuprofen and other NSAIDs (nonsteroidal anti-inflammatory drugs) can get in the way of your healing.[2] Steroids can decrease the tensile strength of wounds and block other aspects of the wound-healing process.[3] If you rely on these drugs to the exclusion of other methods—such as ice and elevation, or acupuncture and magnets (which can help reduce swelling)—you may end up weakening your self-healing potential. Another example is chemotherapy: the drugs used for cancer treatment tend to limit cell proliferation, which is good for knocking out cancer but bad if you also want to support wound healing and healthy immunity. Finding a balance between the positive effects of these medications while limiting their negative effects on wound healing is important.

---

*When we say that anti-inflammatory drugs can impede wound healing, we do not mean to imply that you should leave them out of your postsurgery program of care. Anti-inflammatory drugs play a key role in controlling inflammation; nonetheless, their excessive or prolonged use can interfere with normal healing.

Poor nutrition. For the person who has recently had surgery, nothing beats a fish-and-vegetable stew or some other well-prepared, nutrient-rich meal. All phases of wound healing depend on a sufficient supply of protein, carbohydrates, vitamins, and minerals. On the flip side, poor nutrition certainly limits healing after surgery. Sadly, in many hospitals today, it is not uncommon to see people sitting in bed for days after a major surgery sucking down Jell-O, ice cream, and sodas—and very little else. By not getting good nutrition at a time when they need it most, these individuals are inadvertently hampering their own recovery. Diets that are too low in protein and high in fat can have very troubling consequences, such as an increased tendency toward chronic inflammation and immune dysfunction. Such diets also tend to produce deficits of the very nutrients you need for optimal wound healing, namely, zinc, protein, glutamine, arginine, and vitamins A, E, C, and B complex. (We discuss these nutrients and how to get them in chapters 3 and 4.) It has been our experience over the years that supplementing the diet with these vital nutrients can greatly improve the healing of surgical wounds.

Excessive body fat. Another major impediment to wound healing is being either obese or overweight. (Obesity is clinically indicated by a body mass index, or BMI, of 30 or more; a BMI between 25 and 29.9 indicates that the person is overweight. Your health care provider can tell you where you stand.) Obese people have cardiovascular and respiratory limitations that, in turn, lead to a reduced oxygen supply. Wound healing depends on a steady supply of oxygen to the tissues affected by the surgery. Lack of exercise or movement only exacerbates these effects. These are among the main reasons obese individuals have a diminished ability to heal after surgery.

High blood sugar. Obese people also are more prone to chronic inflammation and chronically elevated blood sugar problems, a disorder also known as diabetes mellitus. High blood sugar levels often delay wound healing and increase the risk of dangerous infections.[4] When blood sugar levels are kept within a moderate range—ideally, between 100 and 140 mg/dL (milligrams per deciliter, the standard unit of measure for blood sugar) around the time of surgery—healing takes place at a faster rate and wound healing problems are less likely.[5] Fasting blood sugar levels in adults should not exceed 100 mg/dL. There is little doubt that a high-fiber diet, regular exercise, and stress management are essential to keeping blood sugar under control. Diet alone—and in particular baked flour products that also contain egg or dairy protein—can be a source of advanced glycation end products, or AGEs, substances that delay wound healing in people with chronically high blood sugar levels.[6]

Physical pain and emotional distress. Pain and anxiety, particularly when persistent and uncontrolled, will unleash a torrent of stress hormones as part of the stress response. Several of these hormones will trigger a constriction of blood vessels under the skin (peripheral vasoconstriction), which then limits the oxygen supply to the surgical wound area. Other stress-related changes can further exacerbate the situation. For example, cortisol and other adrenal hormones secreted during stress tend to dampen the inflammatory response, which again is needed for the second phase of wound healing. In chapter 5, we focus a great deal of attention on ways to help you temper the stress response and overcome its more menacing aspects.

Lack of sleep. Sleep and healing form an intimate partnership, and, indeed, a great deal of healing takes place automatically while you sleep. When your tissues become damaged, the rate of healing is always greater during sleep—regardless of when the surgery or injury occurred.[7] If you don't sleep or take steps to promote deep sleep, your healing process will be markedly delayed after surgery.[8] A stressful day coupled with a restless night can greatly compromise your ability to heal effectively after surgery. We address practical aspects of improving your sleep in chapter 7.

A toxic lifestyle. Pollutants and toxic lifestyle habits like smoking and drinking can further tax the body's wound-healing resources. Of these unhealthy habits, the effects of smoking are by far the best studied. Surgeons have known for decades that people who smoke experience a much slower recovery from surgery. Consider this short list of factors:

- A number of studies of bone and joint fusions (orthopedic surgery) have demonstrated that smokers are far more likely than nonsmokers to experience a failed union, delayed healing, more pain, and increased complications.[9]

- Among breast cancer patients undergoing surgery, smokers were 9 times more likely to develop the wound-healing problem known as skin flap necrosis.[10]
- Smokers undergoing a "tummy tuck" (abdominoplasty) were 3 times more likely to experience wound healing problems before getting out of the hospital compared to the nonsmokers.[11]

So insidious are the effects of smoking that some plastic surgeons actually forbid their patients to smoke after cosmetic and reconstructive operations.[12] Anyone who has seen the wrinkled skin of longtime smokers cannot fail to understand why. It's generally known that having a smoker stop smoking at least 2 days in advance of the surgery, and staying tobacco-free for at least 8 weeks after the operation, can help eliminate many of the postoperative risks associated with the habit.

Studies of patients who have coronary artery bypass help illustrate the value of giving up a smoking habit before and after surgery. After two days of being off cigarettes, the adverse effects of nicotine on the cardiovascular system have disappeared. By the second week, respiratory function has markedly improved, with less sputum or excess mucus, and after 2 months, lung function has returned to near normal. Nonetheless, patients who have a history of smoking more than 20 pack years (one pack a day for 20 years, two packs a day for 10 years) show a much greater risk for complications from the surgery.[13]

What is it about smoking that makes it so bad for the healing process? Much of the blame has to do with three toxins found in cigarette smoke: carbon monoxide (which limits oxygen transport in the blood), hydrogen cyanide, and nicotine.[14] Tobacco smoke actually contains some 4,000 different chemicals, and many of these can contribute to biochemical imbalances like chronic inflammation and oxidative stress, both of which tend to limit wound healing. Smoking also results in a greatly increased risk of surgery-related infections as well as various nutritional deficiencies—which may themselves contribute to the wound-healing problems seen in smokers. We know, for example, that many smokers are deficient in vitamin C.[15] Such a deficiency could get in the way of the wound-healing process, since vitamin C is needed for collagen synthesis and other aspects of tissue repair.[16] Stress and anti-inflammatory medications tend to further tax the body's vitamin C supply.

After you, your surgeon, and health care team remove any roadblocks to your period of healing, the next step is to focus on how to support that process. In the next few sections of this chapter, we'll introduce you to the different parts of your rapid recovery program. Then, in subsequent chapters, we'll go into the different aspects of the program in much greater detail.

✤ Repair-Enhancing Nutrition and Botanicals

Every one of our patients who has had an outstanding recovery from major surgery have had a common denominator: they embraced whatever helped them heal and got rid of, or minimized, anything that got in the way.

Nutrition is the number one tool in the repair toolbox. With optimal nutrition, you can tolerate the stress of surgery because your body has enough energy and a hefty supply of the nutrients that support wound healing. These vital reserves enable you to withstand the metabolic insults and semistarvation states brought on by the surgery. The reserves tend to be low in people who are either too old or too young, and in people who are debilitated or suffering from infections.

When we say nutrition, we're talking about not just diet, but supplements as well—those entirely nontoxic natural compounds that can influence our repair-enhancing biochemistry in many different ways. Among the supplements we will highlight, with specific recommendations for dosage and timing, are vitamins A, B complex, C, and D, as well as zinc, glutamine, arginine, carnitine, melatonin, glucosamine, chondroitin sulfate, and omega-3 fats.

Some of these supplements have more scientific support than others. For the ones that are more scientifically questionable, we offer the appropriate caveats and suggestions for safe use. In some cases, dosages are extremely critical. For example, taking vitamins D and E in high doses can actually impair the wound healing process. Blood-thinning herbs and nutrients will generally need to be avoided in the week prior to surgery and on the day of the operation. Taking these agents close to the time of surgery can increase the risk of heavy bleeding or hemorrhage.

Throughout this book, we also highlight the therapeutic value of various herbal supplements, namely, echinacea, ginseng, astragalus, gingko, goldenseal, bromelain, gotu kola (*Centella asiatica*), milk thistle,, curcumin, Saint-John's-wort, and aloe vera. Some herbals have shown promise when used externally after surgery, including tea tree oil, comfrey, aloe vera, gotu kola, and calendula. These topical herbs can easily be applied as creams or ointments at home, and often bring the same kinds of relief afforded by pharmaceutical preparations.

Depending on the situation, one or more of the above herbs may be recommended. For example, ginseng and astragalus can be helpful in the first two weeks after major surgery, as both herbs have been shown to support the body's resistance to stress. We often recommend these herbs to people who are debilitated or lacking in vitality. Pantothenic acid and other B vitamins, as well as vitamin C, zinc, and bioflavonoids, can bolster your resilience immediately after your operation.

On the flip side, though, it's important to be aware of key caveats for using these supplements. For example, as mentioned earlier, blood-thinning supplements such as vitamin E and feverfew can lead to excessive bleeding or hemorrhage. Some supplements may interact badly with anesthesia. Vitamin E, in cream form, has also been shown to hurt wound healing, apparently because it inhibits the formation of new blood vessels needed for wound healing.

✎ Body-Centered Support

Movement, osteopathic manipulation, massage, chiropractic, physical therapy, and other forms of bodywork are excellent ways to enhance your body's healing potential. Movement supports the wound-repair process by improving blood and lymphatic circulation. This improved circulation ensures that more oxygen and vital nutrients get to the wound area, while toxins are more efficiently removed.

Your physical activity level should be in line with your ability, energy, and overall health. If you have a lot of inflammation because of the surgery, activity should only be gradually increased. Becoming too active soon after the surgery tends to make inflammation worse. At the other extreme, however, lying in bed all day can delay repair because of the important function that movement plays in improving circulation and in alleviating pain. Surgical complications such as deep vein thrombosis (potentially deadly clotting) and incontinence happen more frequently when the patient stays immobile. Research suggests that some degeneration of the joints may even occur within 24 hours of becoming immobile. Even passive movement can have some positive effects in the period right after surgery. The solution, then, is to be mildly but regularly active in the days and weeks after your surgery.

Surgeons routinely recommend that their patients become physically active again as soon as possible after the surgery. Nonetheless, it is crucial that the activity be gentle and gradual in the early phases; this is where walking, stretching, yoga, and other mindful disciplines such as qigong and tai chi have been particularly helpful. In chapter 5, we provide some examples of mindfulness exercises and stretches that will minimize stress on your body in the first few weeks after surgery. Bodywork is an equally important part of physical care. You may find that your physical therapist is the most important member of your recovery team.

Massage therapy also can be helpful. Massage not only enhances circulation but can break up fibrosis to prevent adhesions from forming, loosen up constricted muscle fibers, relieve swelling, and reduce muscular tension. One form of massage, called manual lymphatic drainage, is used to improve the lymphatics and blood circulation; this can be especially helpful for patients who have interrupted blood flow and poor lymphatic function postsurgery.

After any form of injury, osteopathic manipulation, massage, and other forms of manual therapy can help diminish the pain and reestablish one's full range of motion after lesions form. For people who have inflamed areas after surgery, hydrotherapy and cryotherapy (ice massage) can be used in combination with various techniques such as Swedish massage, mild compression, pressure point therapy, cross-fiber friction, and joint mobilization.

Acupuncture, therapeutic touch, Reiki, and other energy-based approaches are among the other bodywork practices that have begun to receive more attention as ways to reduce postoperative pain, nausea, and vomiting, while enhancing energy and healing. Last, hyperbaric (high-pressure) oxygen therapy, whirlpool therapy, electrical stimulation, and magnetic therapy are additional ways to enhance tissue repair. (Though a few of these strategies can be carried out on your own, most require a skilled practitioner and are beyond the scope of this book.)

᷎ Emotional and Psychological Support

Whether you're having minor or major surgery, the experience can trigger feelings of fear and anxiety. This stress response itself can be problematic for the wound-healing process and lead to many surgical complications. The mind-body techniques we will cover will help you prepare for surgery (chapter 5) and then recover more effectively in the sometimes painful aftermath of surgery (chapter 6). Hypnosis, self-hypnosis, and mindful breathing are simple, noninvasive methods to decrease the stress response. Many studies have found that patients who practice these techniques experience less postoperative pain and discomfort, less nausea, better immunity, fewer complications, better energy levels, and significantly faster recovery times overall.[17]

How much you worry just before your operation can have a negative impact on your ability to heal afterward.[18] So, while it may be surprising, simply preparing yourself with a deep relaxation script can save thousands of dollars in hospital bills. Mind-body techniques have consistently been linked with quicker recoveries in clinical studies. These techniques may be particularly helpful for people who have led highly active, independent lives and now find themselves changed or restricted in some way because of the surgery.

Coping dynamics play a vital role as well. For some people, too much detailed information creates anxiety; whereas for others, too little information leads to more worry and tension. Figure out which is better for you. Also important is learning how to confide in others, either individually or in support groups, and having other outlets for emotional expression, such as journal writing and art therapy. Trust your own judgment about the resources available and to find the outlets and pathways that feel most comfortable and supportive to you personally, rather than relying on what others tell you you *should* be doing.

Over the long term, mind-body techniques can be a great way to manage the grief, anxiety, and depression that sometimes linger for many months after major surgery. Grief over losing an organ or a normal physical function—for example, losing fertility after removal of the uterus or ovaries—may call for counseling or emotional work. For many people, the process of long-range recuperation is a matter of exploring spiritual openings, such as gratitude and forgiveness. It's also about cultivating a deeper understanding of life and death, truth and reality, that we often glimpse after squarely facing our losses and crises. And in many cases, it's about becoming integrated into a new way of being and belonging in the world. For many people, using spiritual support such as prayer or meditation helps not only with this integration process but with deepening one's appreciation of life and health.[19] Prayer, whether done by the patient or by others, appears to reduce pain and fatigue and can have a positive overall influence on healing.[20]

Wound Healing 101: A Basic Description of the Process

If you've ever had surgery or a major injury, there's a chance you were struck by a sense of wonder as you thought about the finer aspects of the body's healing process after the operation: how the body, once opened up, managed to close the area without bleeding to death in the interim; how damaged tissues regenerated, eventually closing up the wound; how chemical signals were instantly sent out to immune cells, which then rushed in to defend against potentially lethal microbes; how, after the anesthesia wore off, the pain intensified and then subsided, while the wound area gradually and seamlessly changed from red and swollen to a fairly normal appearance. Eventually, healthy tissues replaced the ones that were damaged, leaving behind little if any trace of the original wound.

How exactly does the body heal from a surgical wound? Wound healing takes place in four basic steps: *wound sealing,* which involves blood clotting and the creation of a scab; the *inflammatory stage,* which involves increased blood flow to and from the wound area; *tissue building,* during which new skin and new blood vessels are formed; and *matrix building,* in which a matrix (mainly consisting of new collagen) is formed for increased strength, stability, and overall integrity. Let's consider each of these briefly in turn, so that you can understand how different interventions might be used to affect each stage.

Step 1: Wound Sealing

With any surgical injury, your body's first challenge is finding a way to slow or limit blood loss. Fortunately, the body is well designed to meet this challenge. For the first 5 to 10 minutes, blood vessels constrict, limiting blood flow to the area. At the same time, blood particles called *platelets* are released from the blood vessel to initiate the clotting process. This prevents blood from leaking out of the damaged vessels.

Blood clotting takes place with the help of a protein called *fibrinogen,* which links up as interwoven strands of *fibrin,* a kind of netting or meshwork. The fibrin and other proteins form a scab or protective covering. This not only prevents the wound from getting contaminated, but also allows cells to move around freely below the surface—another essential part of the wound-healing process. The laying down of this new tissue layer or epithelium (a process also known as *epithelialization*) normally produces a watertight seal within 24 hours.

As noted earlier in this chapter, there are supplements such as vitamin E that can thin the blood and retard the wound-healing process. Later in this book, we'll cover these supplements and their role in blood thinning in detail.

Step 2: Inflammatory Control

After the successful sealing of the wound, blood vessels dilate and blood flow increases rapidly. Now the wound area turns reddish, hot, and swollen. The increased blood flow enables the rapid removal of toxins, dead cells, and debris. This cleansing of the wound must take place to prevent infection, and it must happen before the next stage of wound healing can effectively begin. White blood cells called *neutrophils* engulf the debris along with bacteria that have moved into the area. The increased white blood cell activity usually stops by the fifth day after surgery, but only if the wound is not contaminated. If the activity persists—due to infection, bad nutrition, medication use, lack of oxygen, or perhaps some combination of these factors—it can interfere with the wound-healing process.

Meanwhile, immune cells called *macrophages* are constantly releasing growth factors and other chemical messages that fulfill a variety of key functions: (1) digesting and killing bacteria, scavenging tissue debris, and destroying the neutrophils; (2) stimulating the immune responses to infection; (3) stimulating the formation of collagen and other proteins essential to the formation of new tissue; and (4) stimulating the formation of new blood vessels (angiogenesis), without which the new tissue would never form. Platelets, the blood particles we mentioned earlier, are also secreting growth factors and other substances that aid in the orderly process of tissue repair.

We mentioned how the increased blood flow of inflammation helps cleanse the wound. It also plays another valuable role, that of increasing *nourishment*. With more blood, there is an increased supply of oxygen, vitamins, and other nutrients to cells in the wound area. When inflammation occurs, the wound area is bathed in blood—blood that ideally would deliver a wealth of nutrients. These nutrients are needed for the construction of new tissue and for the healthy metabolism of those cells—notably the fibroblasts—that participate in the next two stages of the process.

Practically speaking, your most important concerns in the inflammatory stage are twofold. First, you want to avoid prolonged or drawn-out inflammation, as this can hamper your healing process. Consuming too much of the omega-6 and hydrogenated dietary fats—from vegetable oils and meats, and from margarine and many processed foods, respectively—will set the biochemical stage for excessive inflammation. Second, you want to avoid blocking the inflammatory response too strongly or abruptly, since some amount of inflammation is needed for optimal tissue repair. Whereas short-term, moderate use of NSAIDs and other anti-inflammatory medications can be helpful, heavy use of these drugs will impede your healing. As much as possible, try to rely on simple techniques like icing and elevation in order to reduce your need for anti-inflammatory drugs. In the next two chapters, we address some key nutritional strategies that will help your body mount a more balanced inflammatory response following surgery.

Finally, some supplements, such as high doses of vitamins D and E, may tend to block angiogenesis, the formation of new blood vessels that is one of the by-products of the inflammatory response. Use of these supplements should therefore be limited in the first two weeks after surgery.

Step 3: Tissue Building

After the initial wound sealing and inflammatory processes there comes the tissue-building stage, where the bulk of tissue repair and rebuilding take place. What we call tissue building entails the growing of new skin and other epithelial tissue through a process called epithelialization. On the outside of the body, the epithelium consists of the skin. On the inside, the epithelium consists of a delicate membrane that lines all of your organs and internal structures. Within the skin, between 3 and 6 hours after the surgical incision has been made, cells called keratinocytes begin to migrate in response to various growth factors and natural chemical messengers—all of which are released in response to the tissue damage. Throughout the tissue-building stage, epithelial cells are migrating and multiplying, and this eventually leads to complete closure of the injured epithelial tissue.

This third stage is also known more technically as the proliferative phase, because new cells and tissues are being formed at a rapid rate. The growth factors generated during the inflammatory stage now stimulate the migration and activation of special cells called fibroblasts. On about the third day after the surgery, the fibroblasts begin to churn out measurable amounts of collagen, and there is a measurable increase in tissue strength by the fourth day. The collagen content increases over the next few weeks, and by the fourth week, about 40 to 70 percent of wound strength has been achieved. In addition to collagen—the raw material of connective tissue—these cells produce other substances essential to wound repair, most notably the glycosaminoglycans.* These substances together form a connective tissue matrix necessary for cell migration and for strengthening the new tissue.

Many of the growth factors at this stage are needed for the creation of new blood vessels—in particular, for the new capillary beds that provide vital nourishment to the newly formed tissues. The blood supply must remain strong in order for fibroblasts to do their work: a lack of oxygen (hypoxia) reduces the mobility of the fibroblasts and disrupts the healing process. Angiogenesis is the formation of new blood vessels. Ironically, it is stimulated by the lack of oxygen that occurs from the disruption of the blood supply when the surgical incision is made.

---

*Probably the best-known glycosaminoglycans are chondroitin sulfate and hyaluronic acid. Others include dermatin sulfate and heparan sulfate.

Step 4: Matrix-Building

The matrix-building stage represents a kind of winding down of the wound-healing process. Doctors and physiologists refer to it as the maturation or remodeling phase, and it can take from 24 days to 2 years to complete. As anyone who has had a major wound well knows, there is a period during which the wound is fragile and can open up again. Robust collagen and other matrix materials are needed to strengthen the tissues newly formed over the wound area. Under healthy or optimal healing conditions, more and more collagen is laid down, reinforcing the matrix of new tissue. The collagen fibers form an increasingly organized lattice structure that, in turn, increases the so-called tensile strength of the wound. If your wound develops a scab, this will detach from the skin and leave new tissue underneath.

As you can see, wound healing involves a series of separate yet interdependent responses to the injury. In the coming chapters, you'll learn about various ways to influence these stages for the better. For optimum tissue repair and recovery, the integrated nature of the wound-healing process calls for a blending of supplements and strategies. In the next chapters, you'll be learning about what foods, nutrients, and botanicals can support each stage.

3

The Nutritional Foundation for Rapid Repair

*I will apply dietetic measures for the
benefit of the sick according to my
ability and judgment: I will keep them
safe from harm and injustice.*

—HIPPOCRATIC OATH

In July 2004, fifty-two-year-old Reah Fischer was rushed to the emergency room for an appendectomy. An infection had spread from her inflamed appendix to her pelvis, requiring two more surgeries just to handle the infection. Between all three events, she spent 15 days in the hospital. "Until then, I'd never really experienced a health crisis," Reah recalls, her sparkling brown eyes growing misty. "They had a tube running down my throat, and they placed me on numerous drugs. They checked my vital signs six or seven times a night, so I had no sleep. It was one of the darkest times of my life. I was in a great deal of pain. I almost died from the stress of it all." And it was about to get even worse.

Two weeks later, Reah felt a lump in her right breast that she says "seemed to have sprung up over night." Results of the biopsy confirmed her fears: she had breast cancer. Analysis of the tumor tissue showed that she had a mutated version of the BRCA1 gene, indicating her potential to develop a more aggressive malignancy. Her oncologist recommended a bilateral mastectomy because of evidence that this type of surgery could significantly prolong survival for women with this particular form of breast cancer.

In preparation for the surgery, Reah invited her daughters and several other close friends, including her rabbi's wife, to join her in a ritual before the surgery. During the ritual, they said Hebrew prayers together, and Reah expressed deep gratitude to her breasts. With the group as her witness, she then wrote a letter to her breasts in her journal and thanked them for all that they had been to her. She later did this for her ovaries as well, sending love to them for her two beautiful daughters. She mourned the loss of all these parts of her body before releasing them, and she made peace with the loss, knowing that it would ultimately enable her to continue enjoying this life.

Reah's ovaries and fallopian tubes came out a few weeks later in order to eliminate the cancer-stimulating impact of estrogen. "For me this operation was easy, really just a blip on the radar screen," she says. "A few days later I almost forgot I'd had the surgery."

The following month, however, Reah underwent plastic surgery in order to have tissue expanders inserted in her chest. This procedure is necessary for women who don't have enough skin and tissue to allow room for an implant after mastectomy. The tissue-expansion process, which takes place over several months, essentially stretches the remaining chest skin to make room for the implant. Nobody had told Reah how agonizing the tissue-expansion process would be, despite the best efforts of her physical therapist and physicians. It's an experience she recalls as "beyond excruciating." When the tissue expanders came out, the implants were put in, and this was the worst surgery of all. Reah had to take morphine and pain meds for several weeks. During this difficult period, she also practiced deep breathing and visualization to help her relax around the pain.

Thanks to the guidance of a holistically minded physician, Reah had maintained a strong nutritional and fitness regimen before coming in for surgery. This included high doses of vitamin C, an antioxidant formula, an aloe vera compound, and two immune-enhancing supplements. Because of the excellent shape she was in, each surgery—the mastectomy and the tissue expansion procedure—took a full hour less than anticipated. There were four drains from her chest area following the surgery, and these had to be changed on an hourly basis. Some women need to keep the drains in for several weeks, but Reah's were out in only one week, when she had her first checkup. Her physician, a renowned plastic surgeon, told Reah that it was the fastest recovery she'd ever seen, and said, "You were in such great shape, it was actually a pleasure operating on you!" Other surgeons had made similar comments about how thrilled they were with the ease with which they could operate on Reah, thanks to her lean, healthy physique.

Every other week, Reah went back to the hospital to have saline injected into the tissue expander. At each visit, she recalls how her physicians commented on the speed with which she was healing, and about the fact that she had had no infections or complications. Two weeks after the mastectomy, Reah had hired a physical therapist, a woman who specialized in assisting with recovery from mastectomy. The physical therapist told Reah that most women need 25 to 30 sessions to return to optimal functioning. Reah had recovered full mobility and integrity in only 8 sessions. During this period, she also received bodywork from someone who performed gentle "energy healing" on her affected tissues, and this provided a deep sense of well-being and connection.

To further support her recovery, Reah attended a nutrition lecture I was giving for cancer survivors and then sought advice from me shortly before her last two operations. Along with her wholesome, low-fat diet, she has taken the Power Healing Drink, an antioxidant-rich multiple, and omega-3 fatty acids for the past year and feels that the regimen has totally transformed her life. Most recently, she was able to get off the sleeping pills that she had required since the multiple operations, and she's sleeping like a baby. With her silvery hair, golden complexion, and radiant smile, Reah is today a walking testimony to the power of this integrative approach to supporting recovery from surgery.

—*MNM*

All surgeons know that healthy people—and *young,* healthy people in particular—heal faster after surgery. This simple-sounding axiom explains why, after undergoing a knee or shoulder reconstruction, the robust soccer player bounces back far more quickly than her deskbound, stockbroker sister receiving the same operation. Then there's the man in his fifties who recovers just as fast from an organ transplantation procedure as a chain-smoking man in his thirties. Clearly, chronological age is not the only way to figure out how efficiently your body can heal a surgical wound. Nor is this efficiency simply a by-product of good genes, positive attitude, or sound medical care.

So what is it about good health that seems to expedite the wound-healing process? The more researchers have probed this question, the more they have come to appreciate the essential role played by good nutrition—the nourishment we derive from wholesome foods as well as from the supplements we take on a regular basis. Our own clinical experience over the years has repeatedly demonstrated that optimizing one's nutrition is the most effective way to speed up wound healing. With the right combinations of nutrients, people simply mend more rapidly, while those on poor diets often never fully reestablish the integrity of their damaged tissues.

⁂ Body Wisdom and the Evolutionary Drive to Survive

The human body is endowed with an astonishing degree of biological intelligence. This intelligence is not limited to the intellect or brain, but actually permeates every single one of the body's trillion-plus cells. Physician Deepak Chopra, in his book *Creating Health,* says the intelligence expresses itself not just at the cellular or tissue level, but also at the sub-cellular or molecular level—within genes, enzymes, cytokines, hormones, and neuropeptides.[1] Collectively, these diverse molecules help orchestrate millions of functions every second of the day, all in a beautifully synchronized manner, and without any effort on our part.

Among the main functions of these natural chemicals is the transmission of information from one cell to another, enabling cells to talk to each other, and allowing the outside world to talk to the whole organism. One of the ways the outside world communicates with the body is through food. Literally tens of thousands of plant-derived chemicals, or *phytonutrients* (also called phytochemicals), flow through the bloodstream after we eat whole grains, legumes, fruits, and vegetables, as well as the animals that eat these foods. These substances are a kind of language for our cells. Nutritional research has shown that phytonutrients trigger responses in our genes and, moreover, increase the communication between cells. Such effects can have a profound bearing on wound healing and immune function. We will return shortly to this point about nutrients "speaking" to our genes; for now, please keep in mind that the foods we eat play an integral role in the information exchange that characterizes the body's innate intelligence.

In relation to wound healing, the body expresses its intelligence by creating order out of disorder—repairing damaged tissues—and in the subsequent restoration of normal function. Over 3 million years, the human body evolved myriad ways to maintain itself in relative harmony, constantly regenerating its own cells and tissues, and functioning within certain dynamic parameters through the complex cellular balancing act we call *homeostasis*. Wound healing is simply another variation on the homeostatic theme. The ability to restore tissue integrity is simply an extension of our built-in ability to maintain biochemical peace and stability.

Most of our patients want to know if they can support their own healing with nutrition. Well, how exactly does nutrition support the wound healing process? During the process of tissue repair, the body must pull together an array of nutrients to form the building blocks for new cells and tissues. Unless these building blocks are provided by the diet, nutrients will be pilfered from vital storage areas such as the muscle, the liver, bone, and other tissues. A prolonged bout of inflammation following the operation can exacerbate the depletion process. For these reasons, then, surgery tends to rob the body of key nutrients, and this explains why extra nutrients are needed both for healing and for helping the body cope with the stress of surgery. We highlight these points when counseling all our surgical patients.

Of course, major surgery *would* pose even more of a threat, were it not for the fact that medical technology has invented numerous ways to ensure your survival. Surgeries that were once considered dangerous are now far safer and more likely to produce the desired outcome. Even after a radical dissection procedure—that is, a surgery involving a deep incision—in which large amounts of blood may be lost, survival is virtually guaranteed because the blood can be constantly replaced in the operating room.

At the time of surgery, however, your body only "knows" one thing at the cellular level: someone or something is cutting into it. A wound is being inflicted. When the skin and tissues within are injured like this, a complex microscopic drama unfolds as the body tries to respond to the physical trauma. In a word, your cells "sense" a threat to your body's survival. The cells have no alternative but to mount what's called the *stress response*. This is the familiar "fight-or-flight" reaction for which we became hardwired after thousands of years of battling and running from saber-toothed tigers and other fierce carnivores.

One possible reason the body responds with fight or flight after a serious wound is that it is all part of the evolutionary drama we faced repeatedly in our more primitive, hunter-gatherer existence: if we were attacked by a wild animal, we had to muster the adrenaline-driven intensity to either fight back or escape, and to do this despite the grim reality that we had been wounded during the encounter. Over time, these experiences helped hardwire the nervous and neurohormonal systems with the wound-healing mechanisms you learned about in chapter 2.

The implications of the body's response to surgery are clear: if you maintain your usual diet and don't take steps to beef up your nutritional reserves, your body becomes depleted in the very materials it needs to mount an effective healing response, and your recovery will not be as smooth as it could have been.

From Paleolithic Sensibility to Modern Maladaptation

The flip side of what we just stated is also true: by optimizing your nutrition around the time of surgery, the limitations mentioned above can be avoided altogether, and the body's intelligence will prevail. This prompts the question: Would our prehistoric ancestors have gained such nutritional support from their diet? The so-called Paleolithic diet followed by hunter-gatherers from 10,000 to at least 40,000 years ago was loaded with wild fruits, nuts, seeds, and vegetables, as well as low-fat wild game. Overall, the diet was low in fat, moderately low in carbohydrate, and high in protein, essential vitamins and minerals, and thousands of antioxidant phytonutrients.[2]

Medical anthropologists and nutrition scientists now believe that the Paleolithic diet of wild plants and animals was the diet for which we modern humans were genetically programmed. S. Boyd Eaton, MD, one of the foremost authorities on Paleolithic nutrition, makes the point that the more you eat like your ancestors, the less susceptible you'll be to inflammatory diseases like arthritis and heart disease.[3] As you'll see in a moment, this has major implications for anyone facing a wound-healing situation.

Before going further, let's address two major misconceptions about the Paleolithic diet as a model for healthy eating. First is the issue of carbohydrate-rich foods. Our culture's fascination with low-carbohydrate, high-protein diets in recent years has led to the popular notion that all carbs are bad—that they can promote weight gain and even degenerative disease. In truth, not all high-carb foods are bad for our health. We may not have evolved on grain products, but we are highly adaptable beings, and whole grains are perfectly healthful foods. They provide us with fiber, vitamin E, and various B vitamins.

It is certainly true, on the other hand, that *refined carbohydrates* like white bread, doughnuts, cakes, and white sugar can exact a heavy toll on our health—including a tendency to promote blood sugar imbalances, weight gain, premature aging, and chronic inflammation. One of the hallmark characteristics of diabetics, people who show chronically high blood sugar levels, is a tendency to have very poor wound healing.[4] Dietary sugars or refined carbohydrates are converted in the body (as well as in baked goods that mix carbs with proteins) to substances called advanced glycation end products, or AGEs; these appear to impair wound healing.[5] These same effects are *not* seen, however, with high-fiber carbohydrate foods like whole brown rice, barley, and oats.

Another common misconception is that Paleolithic nutrition theory sanctions eating large amounts of meat or meat of any kind. Our ancestors were highly active compared to modern-day humans, and thus they would have metabolized the excess protein fairly well. Moreover, the wild game of prehistoric times was low in total fat but relatively high in omega-3 fatty acids, not to mention free of pesticides, synthetic hormones, and other pollutants. With the advent of agriculture and the domestication of animals, the omega-3 content rapidly dwindled. Americans today consume an 11:1 ratio of omega-6 to omega-3 fatty acids, whereas the more ideal ratio, typical of Paleolithic diets, would range from 1:1 to 4:1.[6] In general, wild meat and domestic meat are worlds apart when it comes to nutritional quality.

It turns out that the typical U.S. diet, with its abundance of fatty meats and dairy products, omega-6-rich vegetable oils, refined grain products, and sugary dessert foods, is a recipe for inflammatory disaster. This diet contains fatty acids that provide the biochemical fuel for the fire of chronic inflammation.[7] By eating such a diet for longer periods of time, you create a high degree of inflammatory potential and are more prone to chronic diseases. When a wound is inflicted, then, a chronic inflammatory response is likely to occur, rather than the more benign, acute inflammatory response that's good for wound healing.

In contrast, the Paleolithic diet—or something close to it—appears to be the ideal diet for keeping chronic inflammation in check. For these reasons, and based on our clinical experiences over the years, we believe that the diet for optimal wound healing should indeed follow the Paleolithic pattern—natural, free of hormone and pesticide residues, high in vegetables and fruits, moderately high in protein and omega-3 fatty acids. The only caveats here are that wild game is not critical—cold-water fish will suffice—and you can still enjoy whole cereal grains, in moderation, without ill effect. If you eat meat, try to buy products that are hormone free and certified as organic.

Along these lines, then, adhering to such a plant-centered, omega-3-rich diet today will help the wound healing process for someone who's had surgery. With its high protein and antioxidant power, the Paleolithic diet is just the kind of eating plan you need to get your rapid repair capacities in full swing. (See chapter 4 for lists of food choices that conform to a plant-centered diet; these lists can be used during the first month after surgery. There is no need for calorie counting as long as you stick with these foods. Nonetheless, monitor your weight and, if weight loss persists, use a higher dose of omega-3 supplement as well as calorie-rich supplements. Be sure to consult with your doctor if you suffer from ongoing weight loss after surgery.)

✺ Understanding Your Nutritional Toolbox

At this point, we'd like to introduce you to the key components of what we call your nutritional toolbox. Before surgery, and in the weeks after surgery, certain combinations of nutrients are as crucial for your recovery as the drugs used to relieve pain and inflammation. Some nutrients continue to play a critical role even

Table 3.1. Impact of Dietary Fats on Inflammation

Fatty Acids	Dietary Sources	Overall Effect*
Arachidonic acid	Beef, liver, and other red meats; poultry, dairy products; also derived from many vegetable oils	Strongly *increases* inflammation
Linoleic acid	Corn oil, safflower oil, sunflower oil, soybean oil, and cottonseed oil; nuts and seeds	Strongly *increases* inflammation
Oleic acid	Pure, virgin olive oil; avocados, almonds, sesame oil, pecans, pistachio nuts, hazelnuts, macadamia nuts, cashews	Very mildly *decreases* inflammation
Gamma linolenic acid (GLA)	Borage oil, black currant oil, evening primrose oil	Moderately *decreases* inflammation
Alpha-linolenic acid (ALA)	Flaxseed, canola oil, soy oil, walnuts, almonds, pumpkin seeds, mustard seeds, algae	Moderately *decreases* inflammation†
Docosahexaenoic acid (DHA)	Cold-water fish, wild game, algae, wild plants	Strongly *decreases* inflammation
Eicosapentaenoic acid (EPA)	Cold-water fish, wild game	Very strongly *decreases* inflammation

*In most cases, these oils must be used long-term in order to achieve the desired effects; however, lean individuals who maintain good nutrition often will respond very rapidly. The addition of antioxidants, berries, cherries, and certain herbs and spices can further enhance one's anti-inflammatory program.

†Alpha-linolenic acid will decrease inflammation only if you are able to convert the omega-3 to its more active forms (EPA and DHA). Roughly half the population is unable to carry out this conversion process.

many months after a coronary bypass, joint replacement, or other major surgery. Certain nutrient combinations are important for the simple reason that they provide what drugs can't provide: the nourishment you need to reestablish and maintain the integrity of the repaired tissues. With the proper nutritional support, these new tissues will become stronger and stronger with each passing day.

Your nutritional foundation for healing includes five major groups of nutrients: (1) proteins, (2) fats, (3) carbohydrates, (4) micronutrients, and (5) phytonutrients. Here's how the five major groups comprise the vital core of your nutritional plan for rapid repair:

- **A balanced supply of high-quality proteins**. Every structure in the human body contains protein, and the synthesis of new protein is an ongoing fact of regeneration. If your diet is low in protein, your immune system will be less resilient, hindering your ability to heal after surgery. The wound area will form less connective tissue (namely, collagen), and will be more likely to break open. Exudate or seepage from the wound, as well as the muscle loss from chronic inflammation and inactivity, can result in a loss of as much as 100 grams of protein daily. For these reasons, getting enough high-quality protein from whey, eggs, fish, and poultry is a must in the first few weeks after surgery. We'll address the more practical aspects of your dietary needs in chapter 4.

  Two of the more healthful sources of *supplemental* protein on the market are soy protein and whey protein. Both are available in powder form, to be added to beverages or meals. Soy is, of course, also available as tofu, soy milk, tempeh, and other soy products. Nancy Collins, PhD, a Florida-based dietitian who has written extensively on nutrition and wound healing, notes that soy has been dubbed an "inferior protein" because of its low amounts of the sulfur-containing amino acids cysteine and methionine. Nonetheless, she says, more recent research indicates that a soy-based vegetarian diet can meet the protein needs of someone recovering from a wound.[8] We recommend that you consider soy as one of several major sources of protein, including egg and whey protein. The latter, a by-product of the cheese-making process, is a high-quality dairy protein available in powder form in many nutrition bars and beverages.

One of the main benefits of improving your protein status, particularly when you do so with whey protein, is that it builds your *glutathione* reserves. Glutathione is a substance composed of three amino acids: cysteine, glycine, and glutamic acid. Glutathione is the primary antioxidant in all our body cells, supporting various antioxidant enzymes that protect your cell membranes from the damaging effects of *free radicals*. Without sounding too technical, free radicals are atoms with unbalanced electrons that are unstable, short-lived, and highly reactive. Stable molecules usually contain pairs of electrons. Metabolism and oxygen-consuming exercise can break the bonds that hold paired electrons together and produce free radicals. As they combine with other atoms that contain unpaired electrons, new radicals are created, and a chain reaction begins that harms DNA, mitochondria, and cell membranes. Glutathione helps protect the cell from such damage. Glutathione in your cells also plays crucial roles in both immunity and detoxification, having been shown to detoxify many pesticides, phenols, household chemicals, bacterial toxins, heavy metals, and numerous carcinogens.

- **A balanced supply of high-quality fats**. Fatty acids are the raw materials that can make or break your body's inflammatory potential. All of the inflammatory chemicals in your body are originally derived from fatty acids, and the balance of "good fats" (omega-3 polyunsaturated fatty acids) and "bad fats" (omega-6 polyunsaturated fatty acids) can determine how inflamed your body will get after surgery. A short bout of inflammation is helpful, but if the inflammation is prolonged—and a diet rich in omega-6 fats would promote this tendency—then healing is impaired and pain becomes chronic. A low-fat diet supplemented with omega-3 fats can also influence key hormonal balances, including estrogens and insulin.

  This is yet another area where fish oil, flax oil, borage oil, and other types of essential fatty acid supplements can prove very helpful. Please note that fish oil is generally a more reliable source of omega-3 fatty acid than are the plant oils. Although your body can convert alpha-linolenic acid (ALA, the plant omega-3) to the more active forms, eicosapentaenoic acid and docosahexaenoic acid (EPA and DHA, the animal omega-3s), this is not a very efficient process. Flax seed oil is widely believed to be a quality source of omega-3 fats, but recent studies show that humans do a very poor job of actually utilizing this source.[9] Women are better than men at converting ALA to the more active omega-3 fatty acids, EPA and DHA.[10] In general, flax oil and other plant sources are poor sources of omega-3s. Ironically, vegan diets and other low-fat diets are generally the most deficient in omega-3 fats (including ALA), and thus these individuals are most in need of supplementation with fish oil.[11] Some omega-3 fats (namely DHA) may also be obtained from algae.

- **A balanced supply of high-quality carbohydrates**. Plants transform sunlight into sugars called carbohydrates. These organic molecules are comprised of three basic elements: carbon, hydrogen, and oxygen. By eating these carbohydrates, we can more easily produce energy, which is why athletes will sometimes consume chocolate bars just before a major competition. When carbohydrates are included as part of a mixed meal that also includes plenty of fiber, they provide us with a sustained source of energy. Carbohydrates are also the major initial building blocks for many other biological structures, including fats and proteins.

  As we noted earlier in this chapter, there are good carbs and bad carbs. The bad carbs include refined carbohydrate foods. Refined starches such as white bread, doughnuts, or pastries act like sugar: they cause a spike in blood sugar and insulin levels. It turns out that such blood sugar surges can increase inflammation, suppress immunity, and even help fuel bacterial infections.[12] Refined starches also tend to make people overweight, and that in turn can exacerbate blood sugar and blood lipid imbalances.

  Good carb choices such as whole unground grains like brown rice and barley, and whole-grain products like whole-wheat bread, quinoa, and pasta should be your main sources of carbohydrate. Whole grains are composed of two health-enhancing parts: the outer layer, or *bran,* and the internal embryo, or *germ.* When grains are transformed into refined foods such as white flour and white rice, the bran and germ and all their beneficial nutrients, antioxidants, and other disease-fighting phytonutrients are systematically removed.

At the present time, whole grains make up a scant 5 percent of the dietary carbohydrate consumed by Americans. And yet there are numerous health advantages to substituting whole grains for most of the refined starches now dominating the typical U.S. diet.[13] There is evidence that whole-grain fiber has many beneficial effects on insulin and estrogen metabolism, as well as on digestive health and weight control.[14] Regular consumption of whole grains has been linked with lower rates of cardiovascular disease and diabetes, as well as reduced risk of dying from various types of cancer and an overall decrease in premature death.[15]

Your body expends a tremendous amount of energy in the aftermath of major surgery. Carbohydrates are broken down in the digestive tract into glucose, which helps power the wound-healing mechanisms such as the formation of new blood vessels (angiogenesis) and the generation of new tissue. The best way to get this energy is to consume sufficient amounts of high-quality carbs.

- **An optimal supply of specific micronutrients.** Just how much healing power can you obtain from your diet? Alas, in terms of meeting the micronutrient and phytonutrient requirements for optimal healing, diet alone is not enough. And existing guidelines for healthful eating, such as the "five-a-day" guideline for preventing cancer and other degenerative diseases, fall woefully short of meeting the nutritional needs of a body in crisis. To meet these "emergency" needs around the time of surgery, you may want additional support from dietary supplements and from the superfoods mentioned above.

Certain vitamins and minerals are essential to effective wound healing, especially because they help provide the additional antioxidant power your body needs in the wake of surgery. The lion's share of research in this area has focused on vitamin C. A deficiency of vitamin C results in a weakening of the newly formed tissue in the wound area (proliferation stage). In both animal and human studies, taking additional vitamin C has been shown to accelerate the healing of ligaments and other connective tissue injuries; bone fractures, too, heal more rapidly with supplemental vitamin C. Vitamin E is helpful in the recycling of vitamin C, but too much vitamin E can be detrimental to wound healing. Trace element deficiencies—notably of zinc and copper—can increase the risk of infections and prolong the wound healing process. Vitamin B_5 and other B-complex vitamins are important for handling the stress response, as well as for the support of protein synthesis.

But more nutrients are not necessarily better. Indeed, that kind of thinking can easily backfire, especially with the trace elements, which have a very narrow range of usefulness. While deficiencies of zinc and copper can delay wound healing, excesses of these same elements can be just as detrimental. The same can be said for high doses of vitamins A and D—too much leads to toxicity and a worsening of one's healing potential.

- **An optimal supply of phytonutrients (plant-derived chemicals).** The plant world provides far more than fiber; it also offers up a cornucopia of natural chemicals known as phytochemicals or phytonutrients (from the Latin *phyto,* meaning plant). These diverse substances can influence human biology in numerous ways, such as decreasing inflammation, enhancing immune function, and even regulating hormone levels.[16] A number of phytonutrients found in herbs have been concentrated and made into supplements. Common examples include curcumin from turmeric, catechins from green tea, and silymarin from milk thistle.[17] These natural agents have been widely embraced in Europe, where herbal medicine has a long and successful track record. There is reason to believe that such supplements may help stave off runaway infections after surgery and can reduce the need for antibiotics.

  The two largest groups of phytonutrients, flavonoids (over 3,000 in all) and carotenoids (over 600 in all), also have been made into supplements. It's not always practical to purify them into separate compounds or ingredients. A more sensible approach is to obtain these phytonutrients in the form of food or superfood supplements, whole-food concentrates such as those allow from freeze-dried greens and berry concentrates. These whole-food preparations enable you to exploit the wondrous principle of *synergy* between the different phytonutrients. When two elements work synergistically, their combined effect is far greater than could be predicted by studying them independently. The whole or partially purified extract of a plant offers major advantages over a single isolated ingredient.[18]

An example is the potent antioxidant lycopene, the bright red pigment found in tomatoes. By combining lycopene with several natural antioxidants such as vitamin E, garlic, glabridin (from licorice), rosmarinic acid and carnosic acid (both from rosemary), the ability to combat oxidative stress and inflammation goes up dramatically—indeed, synergistically.[19] As you may recall from chapter 2, controlling these processes is essential to wound healing.

The use of green superfoods also enables you to consume large amounts of beneficial antioxidants in the naturally balanced proportions found in vegetables and fruits. Green superfoods are powdered dehydrated vegetable and/or fruit combinations that are widely available in the nutritional supplement section of stores. These proportions not only take advantage of the synergy principle, but also appear to provide the antioxidants in a safer form than, say, high-dose vitamin C. With the help of these superfood supplements, you can easily obtain the phytonutrient equivalent of 20 to 30 servings of fruits and vegetables per day. Green superfoods supplement your body's antioxidant power—essential for the overall success and speed of wound healing.[20]

Now that you've been introduced to the tools within your nutritional toolbox and the rationale behind their use, let's focus on how they can be used to specifically speed up tissue repair after surgery. This framework will help you understand why certain nutritional strategies will be emphasized more strongly than others at different stages of your wound-healing journey.

✂ Using Nutrition to Accelerate Tissue Repair

To understand how specific foods, superfoods, and supplements can support you through surgery and improve your post-op recovery, it's helpful to think in terms of the four basic stages of wound healing.

1. **Wound-sealing nutrition.** Vitamin K is a key nutrient important for blood clotting, which is vital for wound sealing. It is abundant in leafy green vegetables and is another reason to embrace a plant-centered diet. Some people are unable to mount an effective clotting response because they lack vitamin K. Vitamin K is a natural clotting agent that is synthesized by bacteria in the intestines; antibiotics can impede this normal production. But most cases of vitamin K deficiency are due to either liver disease or intestinal disorders that involve an inability to absorb fat (vitamin K is fat-soluble). If bleeding or hemorrhaging is a concern, your doctor may recommend preventive doses of vitamin K. There is some evidence that coenzyme Q10, which is now being used for treating heart disease patients, has vitamin K–like effects and can have similar blood-coagulating effects. Maintaining good nutrition overall largely ensures that enough vitamin K is produced and that the wound-sealing process proceeds as efficiently as possible

2. **Fire-fighting nutrition.** The inflammatory stage is the first part of the wound healing process and usually lasts from a few days to a week. Inflammation serves to increase blood flow and clear out debris from the wound area—and limit infection in the process. Thus, nutrients and immune factors flow in, while debris and bacteria flow out. A short or acute bout of inflammation, therefore, is a good thing and a natural part of wound healing.

   When inflammation is chronic, however, the immune system becomes depressed and infection becomes more likely; this can further prolong the healing process. (The immune system itself requires adequate nutritional support in the form of a good diet and multivitamin supplement.) At any rate, you can begin to see why chronic inflammation is clearly undesirable. Overuse of steroids can exacerbate the tendency toward chronic inflammation.

The type of diet that can quell inflammation is a diet similar to the one followed by our hunter-gatherer ancestors. This diet, along with anti-inflammatory supplements including fish oil (or an EPA-rich supplement), gamma-linolenic aid (GLA), vitamins C and E, alpha-lipoic acid, N-acetylcysteine, carotenoids, curcumin, bromelain, and boswellia, form the core of the rapid repair program.

Much research has centered on fish oil. Supplementing with fish oil before and during surgery has led to better outcomes such as lower rates of infection and has shortened the hospital stays for patients recovering from surgery.[21]

Unlike drugs, these natural substances do not appear to have any adverse effects—they don't suppress inflammation to the extent that they would limit wound healing, and thus can be used for longer periods of time, at a fraction of the cost.

3. **Tissue-building nutrition.** After the inflammatory stage, the tissue-building stage goes on for three weeks to several months, depending on the severity of the wound. New blood vessels form, providing additional avenues for delivering nutrients and removing toxins. The tissue-building nutrients are those that provide the raw materials or substrates for various types of tissue—for example, bone versus skin or ligaments.

Dietwise, this stage calls for high-quality protein sources. In addition to diet, a number of supplements help support protein synthesis and other anabolic (restorative, regenerative) processes. We cover these supplements in chapters 7 and 8. A number of amino acids have anabolic or tissue-building effects, especially when used in combination. These building blocks of protein can be obtained in supplement form and will support the processes that bolster growth factor production and further accelerate tissue repair. Physical therapy and other body therapies should begin in earnest at this stage. Various trace elements also support protein synthesis, which is why multivitamin and mineral supplements make good sense.

4. Matrix-maturing nutrition. Also known as the maturation and remodeling stage, the matrix-maturing stage lasts up to two years. During this time, new collagen forms, increasing the overall strength and integrity of tissue in the area. In time, the skin around the wound area becomes softer, more pliable, and more resilient. As usual, it's important to be getting enough high-quality protein during this time. Vitamin C, alpha-lipoic acid, bioflavonoids, and other nutrients will be extremely helpful to the completion of this part of the wound healing process. Vitamin C alone has been linked to the increasing tensile strength of wounds, but there are other micronutrients that seem to enhance this effect. The shape and strength that tissues develop is highly influenced by the movement and mechanical forces they experience. Therefore, it is imperative to move, maintain blood flow, and exercise the area that is healing in an appropriate manner.

Fruits and vegetables are a major source of vitamin C, one of the key collagen builders. Among the other supplements for the repair of collagen and other connective tissues are aloe vera, free-form amino acid complex, L-lysine, glucosamine sulfate, chondroitin sulfate, and methylsulfonylmethane (MSM). Keep in mind that among people who have undergone surgery, an inadequate vitamin C supply is the rule rather than the exception. This is especially the case for elderly people, alcoholics, heavy smokers, and undernourished drug users. To make matters worse, the typical American diet is deficient in vitamin C, as well as in other nutrients that play key roles in wound healing—zinc, copper, glutamine, and arginine. Less than 1 in every 10 Americans eats the five servings of fruits and vegetables per day, and these foods are the only source of vitamin C outside of supplements.

At several points in this chapter, we've alluded to the value of nutritional support *after* surgery. Nonetheless, if you have a chance to begin a nutritional program *before* your operation, you can begin to build up your nutritional reserves—especially in terms of the omega-3 fatty acids, which can take several months to build up in your tissues. If you know that you're going in for a major surgery, and you have at least a few weeks to prepare, then you will be in excellent shape to follow the guidelines in this book.

❧ An Integrative Approach to Nutrition

By now we hope we've convinced you that good nutrition is essential for wound healing to take place. If you ignore your nutritional status and eat a typical "hospital diet" of white bread, meat, cheese, and bland vegetables, you will simply compromise your ability to heal and subsequently prolong the wound healing process. It's not enough to avoid the more problematic dietary items such as sugar, beef, corn oil, and alcohol—you need to be proactive and emphasize the anti-inflammatory and tissue- and matrix-building supplements as well.

Most of the research from the brave new world of nutritional therapy comes directly from studies of wound healing in the aftermath of surgery. Remember that many nutrient combinations not only play a vital role in wound healing, but also help to maintain immune competence and decrease the risk of infection. Nutrients like glutamine and various antioxidants can reduce the risk of life-threatening sepsis and other postoperative complications, while also reducing the overall stay in the hospital.[22] The immune-enhancing benefits are particularly critical for older people, for whom post-op infections are a major concern.

A study conducted at Brigham and Women's Hospital in Boston shows just how powerful the use of nutritional therapy strategies can be.[23] Patients who undergo bone marrow transplants are exposed to extremely toxic drugs during and after their procedure, and their immune systems often take a long time to recover. The Boston study evaluated the effect of glutamine supplementation in 43 patients receiving bone marrow transplants. The length of the hospital stay was significantly shorter in the glutamine-supplemented group compared to the control group—shorter by one week on average. For the glutamine group, the rates of clinical infection and microbial cultures were significantly lower.

An even more striking finding was the extent to which these clinical outcomes translated into significantly lower medical costs. Hospital charges—including medical care and room-and-board charges—were a whopping $21,095 less per glutamine-supplemented patient. Clearly, the addition of this simple yet powerful immune-enhancing supplement resulted in major costs savings and clinical benefits for patients subjected to this highly stressful surgical situation. Other clinically proven benefits of glutamine supplementation include a marked reduction in the use of narcotics among surgical patients and the preservation of healthy liver function.[24]

In addition to glutamine and fish oil, the amino acid arginine has been used with some success to counteract the inflammatory complications that sometimes arise in the post-op period.[25] Under normal conditions, the 5 grams a day of arginine found in the typical U.S. diet is just barely adequate to maintain tissue health. Several clinical trials have now demonstrated, however, that in patients undergoing various forms of major surgery, supplementing with 15 to 25 grams of arginine in the week prior to surgery significantly reduced protein losses when compared with patients receiving conventional nutritional support. More important, in each of these studies, taking arginine promoted more rapid recovery and an earlier discharge from the hospital.[26]

With this remarkable research in mind, it may be tempting to fixate on just one or two supplements—say, arginine and glutamine—while ignoring the rest. But larger combinations of these supplements are clearly the way to go. For example, both glutamine and fish oil supplements have been shown to improve protein balance and reduce the muscle wasting that tends to occur after major surgery.[27] Combining vitamin E with fish oil further enhances its anti-inflammatory impact, and combining vitamin E with glutamine makes the latter even more effective in protecting your liver after the toxic rigors of a bone marrow transplant.[28]

These examples help illustrate some of the ways in which an integrative approach to nutrition can determine your wound healing success in the wake of surgery. Although nutrition is not the *entire* basis for one's wound-healing efficiency, it appears to be a highly pivotal, practical factor. We envision a time when using nutritional therapy as an adjunct to surgery will simply be considered good medicine, a time when all surgeons will recognize the profound support provided by specific nutrients and other natural supplements to promote optimum healing.

If you're like most people, you probably feel empowered knowing that you can take specific actions to positively influence your own recovery. By the same token, though, you know that making major changes in your diet and lifestyle can be a hefty challenge. Many people make the mistake of thinking that if they can't get their diet on track, then at least they'll derive some benefit from the supplements. This is fragmented logic, and it misses the boat for the simple reason that diet is the foundation for nutritional healing. If your diet is bad, your supplements will be of little benefit. By making your dietary foundation as strong as possible, you enable your supplements and other aspects of the program to work more effectively.

Now that the basic nutritional building blocks of repair are familiar to you, we will introduce you to the core practical aspects of the rapid recovery program in the next chapter.

4

Prepare to Repair

With the help of a surgeon, he might yet recover.

—SHAKESPEARE,
A MIDSUMMER NIGHT'S DREAM

When Michael B., a fifty-eight-year-old man from the Boston area, came to see me, he had suffered for years from diabetes. He was looking for guidance on how to use nutrition to better control his condition. Blood tests a few months earlier had shown that his glucose and insulin levels were spinning wildly out of control. At the same time, his eyesight was beginning to fade. He had recently begun suffering from recurrent foot infections along with an uncomfortable tingling in his hands and other parts of his body, a condition known as diabetic neuropathy.

By the time Michael called me for advice, he had already undergone three laser surgeries for his eyes (a common diabetic condition known as diabetic retinopathy), and there were clear signs of cardiovascular discord as well: chest pains, shortness of breath, cold hands and feet, and high cholesterol. Compared to the general population, people with diabetes have a much greater risk of developing heart disease and having a heart attack.

I referred Michael to a registered dietitian who lived in his area and specialized in helping people with diabetes. She and I collaborated on a nutritional plan for Michael that included plenty of legumes and vegetables, as well as moderate amounts of protein from fish and small amounts of poultry. We showed him how to use nuts, seeds, olive oil, and flax oil as his primary sources of dietary fat, and we highlighted the benefits of a high-quality omega-3 supplement along with an antioxidant multiple and extra chromium to bolster his blood sugar control.

By this time, Michael's diabetic condition and poor circulation had already made him prone to abrasions and infections in his feet. He had lost one of his big toes to a runaway infection that resulted in the need for amputation. To help him prepare for the second surgery and lower his risk of developing an infection, I urged him to take the Power Healing Drink with extra amounts of whey protein and to increase his use of an antioxidant multiple along with chromium (for blood sugar control), lutein (for his eyes), and alpha-lipoic acid. The latter supplement had been shown to help reduce peripheral neuropathy and other diabetic complications in clinical trials. I also suggested taking a "mushroom mix" for bolstering his immune function. Finally, I had urged him to use weights and a Thera-Band (a rubbery band that can be used for flexibility and resistance training) to strengthen his upper body in order to prepare for walking on crutches after the operation. I also instructed him to follow a simple tai chi sequence that would provide relaxation while gently strengthening his leg muscles.

As a general rule, the postsurgery recovery for people with diabetes is twice as long as that of nondiabetic individuals. The foot surgeon told Michael that based on his recent history and the slow recovery from the first operation, he would likely need about 3 months to fully recover. But Michael's rate of recovery was much faster. He was back to normal functioning within 5 weeks of the operation and never went on to develop another foot infection. Research suggests that Michael's antioxidant-rich diet and supplement regimen may have also helped slow the decline of his eyes, heart, and kidneys—three of the most frequent targets of diabetes. I feel certain that the nutritional and exercise regimen he adopted prior to and following his surgery was instrumental in his recovery.

—MNM

When we think about speeding up tissue repair, we tend to focus on the healing that takes place after the operation, when the body is experiencing the sometimes painful and stressful aftermath of the surgery. But this is only one part of the story. What you do *before* the operation, especially in terms of your daily diet and overall nutrition, has a vital impact on what happens afterward.

In this chapter, we will show you why the preoperative period offers a potent opportunity for shoring up your healing reserves and readying yourself for the challenges ahead. We will focus mostly on the different ways you can use nutrition to strengthen yourself now and improve your recovery later on. Of course, the dietary recommendations can be maintained long after you have had your operation because they support general health and well-being and will help you meet your long-term nutritional needs. At the end of the chapter, we will touch on mind-body and body-centered care issues.

❧ Nutritional and Botanical Tools for Repair and Recovery

Many surgical situations can be taxing, causing a severe drain on the body's resources. By bolstering your nutritional reserves beforehand, you can avoid or greatly reduce most of the more taxing effects of surgery.

The nutritional foundation that will prepare you for the challenges of surgery depends on a balance of *macronutrients* and *micronutrients*. Macronutrients—proteins, fats, and carbohydrates—function in a cooperative way to support the healing process. They supply the energy and raw materials needed for tissue maintenance and repair. Adequate amounts of carbohydrates and fat are needed to provide the energy to preserve protein for forming and maintaining muscle. Micronutrients include vitamins, minerals, and trace elements. Many of these and a myriad of phytonutrients are supplied by the vegetable kingdom. The nutritional preparation we recommend for elective or nonemergency surgery is designed to give your body a decisive edge in the postoperative period. This means filling up with nutrients that give you the greatest possible control over inflammation and oxidative stress. It means having a strong supply of antioxidant micronutrients and phytonutrients as well as a good balance of fats, proteins, and carbohydrates.

This balanced combination of nutrients, micronutrients, and phytonutrients provides the foundation for effective healing. As practitioners of integrative medicine, we know that those of our patients who have adopted a good diet and the use of specific dietary supplements are supporting their healing system in profound ways, as these same patients consistently have exceptional rates of recovery. We also know that it can be very difficult for people to change their habits of eating, and a great deal of focus, willpower, and planning often are needed to transform old patterns. Once the changes have been made, however, the resulting experience of increased vitality and well-being enables the new habits to take root and become an enduring contribution to health.

Practical Guidelines for Healthy Eating

Everyone needs good food, well prepared, for optimal healing. Try to get three nutritionally balanced meals a day. If you're bedridden, your portion sizes may be very small, because your appetite and digestion are likely to be suppressed. Until you become more physically active, you'll need to eat more of the softer, easier-to-digest foods like fish stew, squash and onion soup, whole-grain porridge, and the Power Healing Drink.

Regardless of whether you're active or inactive, however, a typical, complete, healthy meal should have the following components: one or two servings of protein such as fish, bean soup, or stew containing tofu or legumes; one serving of whole grain such as whole brown rice, millet, pearl barley, or pasta; two servings of vegetables, including two or more varieties of green and dark-orange vegetables; and a small serving of fruit, or several servings when you expect to be physically active. In addition, we recommend taking "core" supplements that will give you even more healing potential. Let's look at each of these parts of your diet.

Getting the Protein You Need for Optimal Healing

Protein is the raw material you need the most so that your cells and tissues can repair and rebuild themselves. But it's also essential for maintaining your immune system; moderating blood sugar surges; building muscle; and producing hormones, enzymes, neurotransmitters, and growth factors. If your diet lacks good-quality protein, all of these critical functions tend to decline, and your health and vitality will quickly follow suit. The damaging effects of not getting enough protein become increasingly pronounced as you get older.

Recommendations for protein sources are typically based on animal-food products such as beef, poultry, dairy, and eggs. Nonetheless, research clearly shows that plant sources of protein are adequate when you eat enough of all the different sources. Grains and beans, for example, can be combined to provide all the essential amino acids for adults. There's no need to combine these varied sources of protein at every meal; just make sure that you eat a range of protein-rich foods throughout the day.

On the other hand, eating *too much protein*—a problem that has been referred to as *protein overload*—can be just as worrisome as not getting enough. Protein overload, a common consequence of trying to follow a low-carbohydrate, high-protein diet for long periods of time, can lead to fatigue, bone loss, kidney damage, blood lipid abnormalities, immune dysfunction, arthritis, and even cancer.[1] Thus, while a little protein is good, more is not necessarily better over the long term.

When we talk about the benefits of beefing up your protein supply, we're really referring to one month before to one to three months after surgery, when your body has increased needs for building new cells and repairing tissues damaged by the surgery. So just how much protein do you need for surgery? Your protein needs are determined primarily by the physiological requirements for growth, cell renewal, and tissue repair. The average adult needs only about *20 to 40 grams of protein each day.* But body size and physical activity levels can increase the requirement considerably, and major surgery further increases your protein needs by two- to threefold. In chapter 7, we show you how to appropriately boost your protein supply in the weeks after surgery.

Keep in mind that protein can only be stored in the muscle. Before and after surgery, then, it would be wise to try to maintain or even increase your muscle mass by resistance training and using free weights or weight machines in conjunction with eating more protein. Vigorous exercise increases your body's production of growth hormone, which in turn stimulates protein synthesis in the muscle, thus accelerating the growth of new muscle.[2] Knowing how to maintain or build muscle is important if you anticipate being waylaid or left inactive by your surgery. The longer you're inactive, the more muscle you'll tend to lose. Building up muscle beforehand with a combination of increased protein intake and resistance training provides a kind of buffer against losing muscle after your operation. This can have more than cosmetic effects: if you lose too much muscle postsurgery, you may then begin to lose protein from other more vital areas—such as the immune system and intestinal tract—and you may fall prey to bothersome infections that further hamper your healing process.[3]

Lunch should be your highest protein meal of the day. Table 4.1 lists the healthiest protein sources for long-term use. Others not listed here include eggs, free-range poultry, and hormone-free, grass-fed beef. These are best used occasionally.

Here are some simple cooking suggestions for preparing beans. Most whole beans (but not lentils) should be soaked for 3 to 5 hours before cooking. Cook beans with a small pinch of sea salt and piece of kombu or alaria (or some other sea vegetable) to reduce gas, enhance digestion, and add minerals. When eaten with grains, take a smaller portion of beans. It is usually best to eat the grains first, then the beans. Many people also benefit from taking a digestive enzyme with dishes that contain beans—a supplement that you can purchase from your local health food store.

Nuts and seeds are also good sources of protein. Due to their lower oil content, seeds are preferable to nuts for daily consumption, and may be lightly roasted and seasoned. Homemade snacks generally are of better quality and preferable to commercial snacks, which should be eaten less frequently.

These healthy sources of protein can readily meet all your needs. Any one or combination of these foods should be included in your daily meals and snacks in the weeks leading up to your surgery. Then continue eating them in the weeks and months after surgery. Whey protein powder in a drink (see page 73) is another excellent way to get protein when you don't have time to cook or need an extra boost. Undenatured (uncooked or unheated) whey protein is most digestible when provided in *hydrolyzed* form, essentially a predigested form of the protein. The one drawback is that this process removes the glutamine, which is a valuable component of whey. Make sure that your whey protein supplement has the glutamine already added back in.

If you have further questions about protein balance in your diet, a registered dietitian can help you determine quantities of food or food portions that may be appropriate for your daily energy expenditure, which roughly corresponds to how physically active you are. Remember, though, that you want to focus not just on *quantity* but *quality* as well. Choose your foods wisely, keeping in mind that some

Table 4.1. Healthy Protein Sources for Daily Use

BEANS

Adzuki beans	Split peas
Lentils (green, red, yellow)	Great northern beans
Chickpea (garbanzo)	Mung beans
Black turtle beans	Lima beans
Pinto beans	Black-eyed peas
Kidney beans	Navy beans
Traditional soy (tofu, tempeh, miso)*	Butter beans

*We recommend reserving the more processed soy products (soy milk, soy burgers, soy cheese, and soy ice cream) for occasional use only.

FISH AND OTHER SEAFOODS

Sole	Carp	Haddock
Salmon	Cod	Herring
Flounder	Trout	Sardines
Halibut	Catfish	Grouper
Scrod	Smelt	Bluefish
Shrimp	Small dried fish (iriko)	Tilapia
Crab	Snapper	Oysters, mussels (fresh)

HEALTHY PROTEIN SNACKS

Seeds	*Nuts*	*Snacks*
Sesame	Almonds	Protein bars ("health bars")
Sunflower	Walnuts	Rice cakes with nut butter
Pumpkin	Pecans	Crackers with hummus
Flaxseed	Filberts	Crackers with goat cheese

protein-rich foods—especially those listed in Table 1—will support your vitality better than others.

Getting the Fat You Need for Optimal Healing

Getting the right kinds of fats in your diet is crucial for controlling inflammation and restoring tissue integrity and health over the long term. Avoid or minimize your consumption of the so-called bad-fat sources: corn oil, sunflower oil, safflower oil, and hydrogenated oils (also called trans-fatty acids, of which margarine is the classic example). The vegetable oils we just mentioned are high in omega-6 fatty acids, notably linoleic acid. These oils should be avoided since they can increase your body's penchant for chronic inflammation, and research suggests that surgical patients in particular should stay away from them as much as possible.[4]

Heating oils causes them to oxidize and undergo other undesirable changes. For this reason, try to use cooking oil only a few times a week at most. For high-temperature cooking such as frying and baking, use coconut oil and palm kernel oil. For moderate cooking such as vegetable sauté, use canola or sesame oil. Olive oil is best reserved for raw consumption, as on salads or with bread.

Maintain a low-fat diet as much as possible. To do this, skip the rich foods like ice cream, cheese, cake, butter, pork, and hamburgers. Please note that most low-fat diets are deficient in omega-3 fats; this is why we emphasize taking a fish oil supplement. Limit the amount of red meats you eat as well as dairy products, with the exception of yogurt. When you do eat red meats, try to select hormone- and antibiotic-free meats and eat them in moderation. Remember that fatty meats tend to concentrate more environmental pollutants, which can damage your health over the long term.

If you eat freely from the foods listed in Tables 1, 2, and 3, you will follow a low-fat diet. If you do have a hankering for fatty fare, try to focus on those foods that contain omega-3 fatty acids, namely cold-water fish, flaxseed, walnuts, and pumpkin seeds. Keep in mind, though, that supplementation with an omega-3 fatty acid will likely be necessary to build up your omega-3 reserves to an optimal level.

How Omega-3 Supplementation Helps You Prepare for Surgery

With the omega-3 fatty acids, we have a simple yet dramatic example of how many of our patients have benefited from nutritional preparation for surgery. Those of our patients taking omega-3 supplements seem to heal up much faster, with less pain and scarring, and they seem to return to work days sooner than others do when on medical sick leave for a given operation. In a word, taking an omega-3 supplement can greatly reduce the inflammatory fallout of major surgery.

Fish oil is the only truly reliable source of eicosapentaenoic acid, or EPA, the omega-3 fatty acid with the strongest anti-inflammatory impact. Ideally, you should supplement with high-quality fish oil at least a few weeks prior to surgery.* The goal is to build up the body's reserves of omega-3 fatty acids while lowering omega-6 levels. The omega-6 fats, which come from land-animal products (beef, cheese, ice cream, etc.) and many vegetable oils, are the essential "fuel" for your body's inflammatory cells.[5] A surplus of omega-6 fats in your tissues is the nutritional basis for runaway inflammation following surgery.

By taking an omega-3 supplement and lowering your body's omega-6 to omega-3 ratio, you will substantially reduce your inflammatory potential—and limit the possibility of having chronic inflammation after the operation. This also ends up lowering your need for potent anti-inflammatory drugs that may ultimately harm rather than help your healing.

Research clearly demonstrates that taking fish oil *before* the operation confers a stronger benefit than taking it *afterward*.[6] Consider the findings from a study by Dr. Evangelos Tsekos and colleagues at an intensive care unit (ICU) in Munich, Germany. All 249 patients in the study had elected for major abdominal surgery and received nutritional support while in the ICU. The first group—considered to be the *control*, or comparison, group—received standard nutritional care, but without fish oil. The second group received standard care along with fish oil after the operation, while the third group received their fish oil *before* the operation. Only this last group of ICU patients who received omega-3s preoperatively showed significantly faster recovery and a shorter hospital stay compared to the first group.[7]

----

*Nordic Naturals is a company that specializes in processing techniques that yield the highest quality omega-3 supplements on the market today. The company extracts and encapsulates the oils under *oxygen-free conditions* in order to avoid oxidation (omega-3s oxidize immediately upon exposure to air). It should also have undergone *molecular distillation*, a process that removes all the heavy metals and other impurities. When you take omega-3 supplements, be sure to follow them with a meal; people over age fifty should consider the use of digestive enzymes to further enhance the effects of these omega-3 fats.

Remember that it takes time to build up your body's reserves of omega-3 fatty acids. If your supply is low—and this is invariably the case if you've been following a typical American diet that includes plenty of red meat, poultry, fried foods, and dairy products—you need a few weeks, at a minimum, to build up your omega-3 supply. Make sure to cut out those foods since they will substantially reduce the benefits you get from omega-3 fats. Your body weight will affect how much of the omega-3 supplement you take and how long you take it. Overweight people naturally need a larger dosage and more time than lean individuals for the simple reason that they have more body fat to replace. (This is also one of the reasons obese individuals frequently show inflammatory imbalances—their body fat is itself the source of a considerable amount of low-level inflammation.) We find that obese individuals typically require several months to replete their body's omega-3 levels. Fish oil, algae, and some land-plant sources are abundant in omega-3 fatty acids. Overweight people should generally take 6 grams per day for 3 months prior to surgery. Thin people can take 3 grams per day, while people of medium weight can take 4 to 5 grams per day. Stop ingesting fish oil one week before surgery. You can then start taking it again 3 days after surgery. (Remember that fish oil is a more reliable source of omega-3 fatty acids compared to flax or flaxseed, because not everyone can convert the plant omega-3s into the active forms of omega-3 fatty acids. Also, see the footnote on page 69 for the best fish oil to use.)

Getting the Carbohydrates You Need for Optimal Healing

Dinner and lunch should be your main carbohydrate-rich meals of the day. We give thumbs up to whole-grain pastas as well as long-grain brown rice, pearl barley, barley, quinoa, millet, and rye berries (which can be cooked with rice). Pressure cooking the grains helps make whole unground cereal grains taste sweeter and also makes them more digestible.

Organically grown cereal grains are always preferable. Although all types of grain are members of the same botanical family, they are not interchangeable in terms of their culinary characteristics or physiological effects. In this regard, note that most of the occasional-use grain products in Table 2 have a fairly high glycemic index. The glycemic index (GI) is a ranking of foods based on their impact on blood sugar levels. Carbohydrate foods that break down rapidly during

Table 4.2. Healthy Carbohydrate Sources

WHOLE GRAINS AND GRAIN PRODUCTS

Regular Use*	Occasional Use
Whole brown rice (long grain)	Sourdough rye bread
Barley	Whole-wheat bread
Pearled barley	Somen and other Asian noodles
Rye (whole rye berries)	Corn tortillas or grits (unless allergic)
Buckwheat (kasha)	Millet
Quinoa	Basmati rice
Wild rice	Brown rice noodles
Oats, oatmeal	Couscous
Bulgur	Unleavened whole rye bread
Amaranth	Sprouted grain bread
Whole grain pastas (thick)	Sweet rice
Whole-grain spaghetti	Rolled oats and rye flakes
Protein-enriched spaghetti	Wheat (unless allergic)
Fettucine	Corn (unless allergic)
Vermicelli	Pumpernickel bread
Angel-hair pasta	Gnocchi
Buckwheat (soba) noodles	Whole-grain English muffins
Sprouted whole-grain/seed breads	

*"Regular use" means every day. "Occasional use" means one to three times a week.

digestion have the highest GIs—that is, their blood sugar response is fast and high. Carbohydrates that break down slowly, releasing glucose slowly into the bloodstream, have a relatively low GI. Rather than fixate on the specific GI value of whole grains and grain products, we ask you to follow these guidelines.

- Stay away from white flour products, candy, and sweeteners. In addition to their high GI ranking, these foods are bereft of nutrients, so it's a bit of a misnomer to call them foods in the first place.

- High GI beverages (e.g., fruit juice), fruits (e.g., watermelon, pineapple, or cantaloupe), and desserts (e.g., cakes or soy ice cream) generally should not be eaten on an empty stomach. Try to consume these foods *after* you've had a mixed meal that contains whole grains, vegetables, and legumes. Indeed, high-GI grains are not a problem when you combine them with beans in the same meal.

- Most breads and baked goods have a high GI. Breads come in many different forms, and generally the heavier whole-grain breads or coarse European varieties are a better choice—they contain ample amounts of fiber and will have an even more benign effect when combined with protein (e.g., turkey or fish) or healthful spreads such as hummus or baba ghanoush (an eggplant spread).

- Noodles and other pastas tend to have a low GI relative to other grain products, and again, eating them with proteins and vegetables will further improve the blood sugar response.

Eating low GI foods will support your energy throughout the day. High GI foods can provide a rush of energy because they produce a big surge in blood sugar levels. In response, however, your body pumps out insulin to quickly remove the excess sugar from your blood. The result is the well-known "crash" phenomenon that follows a sugar binge: the energy "high" is invariably followed by an energy "low" when you eat high-GI foods. Eating foods with low glycemic values* will keep you from getting caught up in this roller coaster of energy highs and lows. Remember that if you do eat high-GI foods, try to combine them with pro-

---

*Another way to gauge the glucose-raising effects of food is the glycemic load. This concept takes into account the blood-glucose-raising effect of the *amount of carbohydrate* consumed—in essence, it simultaneously describes the quantity and quality (glycemic index) of carbohydrate in a meal. You calculate the glycemic load of a food by multiplying the glycemic index by the grams of carbohydrate in a food and dividing the total by 100. Each unit of the glycemic load represents the equivalent blood-glucose-raising effect of 1 gram of pure glucose or 1 gram of white bread.

teins (especially legumes) and fiber-rich foods to temper the blood sugar response. Your blood sugar levels—and thus your energy levels—will remain more stable, balanced, and harmonious throughout the day.

Eat Your Vegetables, Savor Your Superfoods

For vital nutrition and fiber, it is important to include two meals daily that contain a hearty amount of vegetables. Emphasize variety throughout the week: kale, collards, cabbage, chard, Brussels sprouts, carrots, onions, radishes, and broccoli are all excellent for regular consumption, and should be lightly steamed to enhance their digestibility. Raw salads are preferable when consuming a high-protein lunch or dinner. Also try eating more sweet-tasting vegetables—cooking squash, daikon radish, and whole onions will enhance their sweetness. Check out new cookbooks for motivation and inspiration.

The Power Healing Drink will help you get more of the phytonutrients from vegetables into your body without having to cook too often. It's a great way to start each day. Here are the ingredients.

> *1 to 3 tsp of green food concentrate*
> *1 scoop of whey powder (hydrolyzed, with glutamine)*
> *1 glass of water or drinkable low-fat yogurt*
> *splash of fruit juice (for added flavor)*
> *1 capful of aloe vera concentrate*

Begin by adding a rounded tablespoon or heaping teaspoon of a green powderized vegetable concentrate (also called a green food) in a glass in water. Add one scoop of whey protein. Add water and a touch of fruit juice for taste, stirring as you add. Add one capful of aloe vera concentrate to the glass. Blend together and enjoy.

Aloe vera enhances wound-healing ability, immune function, gastrointestinal integrity, and digestion. Discontinue aloe vera one week before surgery, though, to avoid excess bleeding and interactions with anesthetic agents. Whey protein, which is rich in sulfur-containing amino acids like *cystine*, enhances your antioxidant power, immune function, and lean-tissue maintenance.[8] Green foods provide a high concentration of numerous antioxidants as well as chlorophyll, which helps to eliminate harmful bacteria, promotes skin repair, transports oxygen, and supports healthy intestinal functioning.

We've been continually impressed with the healing benefits people report after trying the Power Healing Drink on a daily basis. One patient of ours, John W., had a recurrent abscess that kept coming back every few months for several years despite drainage and antibiotics. He started using the drink before and after his last surgery and has been abscess free for the past three years. Other benefits he observed included better energy levels throughout the day and a steady improvement in his skin and joint health.

According to the National Institutes of Health, to get the amount of phytonutrients we need for maximum protection against degenerative diseases, we should be eating at least 10 servings of vegetables and fruits daily. This is quite a contrast from the "five-a-day" guideline put forth by the American Cancer Society. The latter advice assumed that nobody could possibly consume, let alone prepare, 10 servings per day. With the introduction of green food concentrates—or what nutritionists now call *superfoods*—we can practically obtain the *phytonutrient equivalent* of 10 to 20 servings a day. This makes the Power Healing Drink a perfect complement to a healthy diet.

Green foods tend to accelerate detoxification processes; thus, various reactions may occur with consistent or increased use of these products. For some individuals, these can include skin rashes, and even fatigue. These are temporary reactions that normally subside in a short period of time. If you have one of these reactions, you might benefit from reducing your dose of the green foods to a level teaspoon for a few days to a week, then gradually increasing it. Your skin appearance will rapidly improve after this. Pregnant women should generally take small or moderate doses of green drinks in order to avoid a detoxification response. Note that most green food products do not contain fiber, which you obviously need for many reasons. Whole grains, fruits, and vegetables should ideally form the core of your diet.

The Power Healing Drink constitutes a highly digestible form of "food" and should not be taken on the day of surgery. Generally speaking, you will be asked to fast on the morning of surgery. Follow your doctor's guidelines for not eating or drinking on the day of your operation. These guidelines will vary depending on the type of surgery, but most surgeons and anesthesiologists require that you take nothing by mouth for 8 hours before surgery. In some cases, you may be asked to avoid foods and beverages the evening before the surgery. Avoiding all food and drink for 8 hours will assure the stomach is completely empty and will help prevent problems with anesthesia, vomiting, and breathing. Most medications can still be taken on the morning of surgery, just with small sips of water, but check with your physician first.

After the surgery, you can return to the Power Healing Drink, making it a morning ritual. Remember that the benefits are incremental and will accrue over time.

Some purists may argue that the whole vegetable is far better than the processed vegetable matter one finds in a so-called green superfood or green powder concentrate. We are not advocating the use of these concentrates as a *substitute* for vegetables; they should instead be viewed as a complement to your diet, providing your body with an easy-to-digest, phytonutrient-rich treat, in the quick-and-easy form of the Power Healing Drink.

Supplementation before Surgery

We recommend certain *core supplements* that everyone can take to help with repair and recovery. Here's an example of how your intake of certain micronutrients before surgery can set you up for rapid repair after the operation. Researchers in Spain measured the preoperative blood levels of zinc and other nutrients in 97 patients who were to receive hemiarthroplasty for an arthritic, degenerated hip.[9] (Also known as arthroplasty, this is a procedure in which the diseased parts of the hip joint are removed and replaced with new, artificial parts.) The investigators then analyzed the various nutritional parameters with respect to how quickly each patient healed from the surgery. There was a highly significant relationship between serum zinc levels and delayed healing in the postoperative period: patients with low zinc levels (below 95 mcg/dL) were *12 times more likely to have delayed healing* compared to patients with normal blood levels. Simply

Table 4.3. Reaping Benefits from the Vegetable Kingdom

VEGETABLES

Regular Use*			Occasional Use
Leafy	**Above Ground**	**Root**	
Collards	Broccoli	Carrot	Water chestnut
Kale	Brussels sprouts	Burdock	Sweet potato
Watercress	Cabbage	Daikon	Yams
Bok choy	Wax or yellow beans	Lotus	Okra
Wintercress	Cauliflower	Rutabaga	Gourd
Mustard greens	Chinese cabbage	Turnip	Escarole
Swiss chard	Celery	Onion	Zucchini
Parsley	Scallions	Parsnip	Bamboo shoots
Dandelion	Leeks	Garlic	Plantain
Rapini	Fresh string beans	Radish	Eggplant
Endive	Chives	Jinenjo	Fennel
Lettuce (fresh)	Fresh green peas	Dried daikon	Rhubarb
Turnip greens	Squash (all kinds)	Dried lotus	Purslane
Kohlrabi	Pumpkin	Dandelion root	
Spinach	Hokkaido pumpkin	Salsify	
Carrot greens	Celeriac	Shallot	
Knotweed	Cucumber	Potato	
Lamb's-quarters	Snap peas	Beets	
Miner's lettuce	Green/red peppers		
Curly dock	Chanterelle mushroom		
Nettles	Shiitake mushroom		
Radish greens	Portabella mushroom		
Bean sprouts	Avocado		
Alfalfa sprouts	Tomato (cooked)		

*"Regular use" means every day. "Occasional use" means once or twice a week. Remember to select your foods with an eye toward freshness. Try to eat a variety of these foods. Most of the occasional-use vegetables contain certain substances that can deplete the body of minerals or have other undesirable effects with regular consumption.

getting enough zinc, then, can support better healing if you're facing surgery for bone fractures and probably for other types of surgery as well.

- **Multivitamin supplement.** This is one of those "nutritional insurance policies" that can be an important way to improve your nutritional status before surgery. Look for a balanced and fully absorbable multinutrient supplement that satisfies your daily requirements for vitamin A (as beta-carotene), vitamin B_1, vitamin B_2, vitamin B_6, vitamin B_{12}, vitamin C, vitamin D, vitamin E, vitamin K, niacinamide, folic acid, pantothenic acid, iron, copper, chromium, zinc, selenium, and magnesium. There are many multivitamins to choose from. Be wary of supplements that claim to be the best multivitamin—these often use cheap, synthetic ingredients, including fillers and additives that can greatly diminish the effectiveness of the multiple. Try to select supplements produced in pharmaceutical *GMP*-(good manufacturing practices) compliant facilities, as these companies adhere to rigorous manufacturing standards that translate into high-quality supplements. Examples include Jarrow, Metagenics, Natural Factors, New Chapter, and Thorne Research. Finally, many enzymes and herbs can greatly enhance the efficacy of vitamins. This is why the best multivitamin supplements contain a scientifically formulated balance of vitamins, minerals, herbal extracts, enzymes, and phytonutrients. Unless the supplement is scientifically formulated, it will likely have poor bioavailability, meaning that most of the ingredients will simply pass through your body with no benefit.

- **Vitamin C**. This vitamin is vital to the smooth healing of tissues. If your multivitamin does not provide at least 1 gram (g) of vitamin C, then take additional vitamin C to ensure that you obtain 1 g daily. Calcium ascorbate, magnesium ascorbate, and ascorbyl palmitate are all good forms of vitamin C, and some supplements provide all three. We urge you to take additional vitamin C in the four weeks leading up to your surgery: 1 to 2 g per day on sedentary days, and 3 to 4 g per day on days when you are physically active. Spread the dose out over the course of the day, 500 mg each time. Use only the buffered form of vitamin C, one that contains bioflavonoids. Stop taking extra vitamin C 7 days before surgery. People with iron overload (hemosiderosis or hemochromatosis), glucose-6-phosphate dehydrogenase deficiency, or kidney problems should consult with their health care practitioner before taking high-dose vitamin C. People with a history of kidney stones should generally not take more than 1 gram per day of vitamin C for extended periods.

- **Vitamin A**. We need this vitamin for tissue development, a healthy immune system, and wound healing.[10] There is now substantial evidence indicating that taking extra vitamin A can benefit people undergoing surgery.[11] Along with aiding tissue repair, vitamin A reverses the steroid-induced inhibition of both superficial and deep-tissue wound healing.[12] This is important because steroids, which are often used after major surgery to help control inflammation, not only delay wound healing but also raise the risk of infection and can cause dehiscence of surgical wounds, a premature bursting open or splitting along the surgical suture lines. Moderate doses of vitamin A (15,000 international units [IU] per day) may help prevent the antihealing effects of prednisone and other corticosteroids.[13] Topical vitamin A may be used in such cases, however, so as not to reverse the therapeutic effects of the corticosteroids. A higher dose of 25,000 IU per day is recommended before and after surgery for people who are poorly nourished or who show gastrointestinal dysfunction.[14] Your multivitamin will already contain some vitamin A, so if you add more vitamin A, try to stay within the 25,000 IU limit. Vitamin A is a fat-soluble vitamin, which is why you need to take it with food. Any extra vitamin A not used by your body right after ingestion is stored in your body fat and liver, to be made available when you need it later on. *Important note*: Vitamin A can be toxic at higher doses; the vast majority of toxicity cases have occurred in the range of 50,000 to 100,000. A daily dose level of 25,000 IU appears to be safe for most adults. Caution must be used when taking vitamin A supplements in situations where the anti-inflammatory effects of steroid drugs are critical, as in organ transplantation. Pregnant and breast-feeding women and people with liver damage should also avoid the higher doses of vitamin A. If in doubt, consult with a nutritionist on this issue.

- **Zinc**. This important trace element stimulates tissue healing and proper connective-tissue formation, and increases the transport of Vitamin A from the liver to the skin, helping to protect body tissue from damage and repair any damage present. It is best to take zinc as part of a balanced multiple. But if the multiple you're taking does not provide at least 15 mg of zinc, then take additional zinc to obtain up to 45 mg per day.

- **Selenium**. Selenium deficits can lead to wound-healing problems. Your multiple should provide between 100 and 200 mcg of selenium. The safe upper limit for adults is 400 mcg—if you exceed that level, you may experience fatigue, nausea, and diarrhea. It's best to not exceed 200 mcg daily.

If you are facing a major surgery that will involve extensive tissue repair or a recovery period of six weeks or longer, we recommend that you consider the addition of zinc and selenium on top of the core supplement regimen. Keep in mind, though, that many antioxidant multiples also contain zinc and selenium.

- **Antioxidant multiple**. As discussed in chapter 3, increasing your antioxidant power is an integral part of your rapid recovery program. We encourage all our patients to start taking an antioxidant multiple in the weeks prior to surgery, and continuing it for several months afterward—especially for people who've had major surgery. This supplement can be taken in combination with the multivitamin and will help provide additional protection against oxidative stress. Look for a balanced antioxidant formula that contains three or more of the following antioxidant factors: alpha-lipoic acid, coenzyme Q10, bilberry fruit extract, lycopene extract, L-carnitine, broccoli powder extract (flavonones), N-acetyl cysteine (NAC), green tea catechins, and grapeseed extract (proanthocyanidins). These antioxidants work within your body at the molecular level, entering the cell and attaching themselves to free radicals found within the confines of the cell. By taking at least three of them, you can take full advantage of the synergies that exist between these antioxidants. The alpha-lipoic acid may be especially important, because it helps preserve and recycle other antioxidants such as vitamin C. One animal study found that alpha-lipoic acid prevented the suppression of wound healing that resulted from excessive doses of essential fatty acids.[15] Try to take this antioxidant multiple once or twice a day in the month prior to surgery and continuing it for three months after surgery.

Our patients—especially those over sixty-five years of age—really seem to benefit from antioxidant support, no matter what type of surgery they're having. Aging tends to load the body with oxidative stress, and surgery certainly increases that unruly burden. A good antioxidant multiple can provide a helpful buffer against both sources of biologic duress. One eighty-five-year-old patient of mine who regularly used such a multiple in addition to a healthy diet was able to leave the hospital one day after major pelvic surgery—indeed, I worked hard to convince her to stay even that long. Only 3 weeks later, she and her husband were off on an exciting cruise down the Amazon.

Other Dietary Tips for Supporting Your Recovery

- Try to emphasize variety in your diet. Variety is better for you nutritionally and for your digestive health.

- Try to buy your groceries at natural food stores or health food stores whenever possible. If you shop at the supermarket, select the freshest foods possible.

- Check the labels on your packaged or canned foods, and avoid or minimize your exposure to food additives such as flavorings, colorings, stabilizers, and preservatives. Try to buy organically grown vegetables and fruits.

- Keep alcohol intake low or moderate—a glass of red wine on occasion, but not on an empty stomach. You should generally avoid all alcohol for one day before and at least 2 weeks after major surgery.

- For improved digestion, make sure your environment is as calm and peaceful as possible; chew your food slowly, turning it to liquid in your mouth before swallowing.

- The use of bitters and digestive enzymes may also be very helpful for digestion. Digestive enzymes are taken with meals and contain pancreatic enzymes such as pancreatin and lipase. These preparations are now widely available in health food stores. Digestive bitters are bitter herbs that stimulate certain taste receptors on the tongue, promoting a reflex secretion of gastrin in the stomach. In Western herbal medicine, bitters have been used to assist with digestion and as a remedy for indigestion (dyspepsia), gastric reflux, heartburn, nausea, vomiting, and loss of appetite.

- If digestive problems persist, such as pain in the abdominal area after eating, you may have food allergies. A specialist can check these for you.

- Do not take any of the above supplements on the day of surgery. And remember to avoid fish oil, vitamin E, high-dose vitamin C, and most herbal supplements during the week before surgery.

- Wait until you begin eating solid foods before taking a multivitamin or fish oil; but it's okay to begin taking the vitamin C and whey protein (which can be part of the Power Healing Drink) even before starting with any solid foods.

- If you notice any bloating or digestive discomfort, you may need to take a digestive enzyme along with the fish oil.

By starting your diet before surgery, you will reap the healing benefits early on, and it will be easier for you to maintain the diet afterward. The diet and supplement guidelines in the preceding pages represent our core nutritional recommendations for your rapid recovery program, to be taken before and after elective surgery. Further adjustments can and should be made depending on your specific surgical circumstances. As we discuss in chapter 8, for example, supplementation with coenzyme Q10 is recommended for patients facing surgeries that affect the heart, lungs, and abdominal area. For people facing orthopedic surgery such as joint reconstruction, glucosamine sulfate and chondroitin sulfate are recommended. It may be helpful to consult with a health care professional for further guidance and tailoring to your particular needs.

❧ Preparing Your Physical Body: Fitness and Muscle Work

Like a runner preparing for a major race, if you're facing surgery, you should get yourself in the healthiest, most robust shape possible before the big event. This is particularly true if you're about to undergo *major* surgery. Nevertheless, some amount of preparation may be helpful even with a relatively minor operation.

Resistance training, using weights or weight machines, is an important aspect of preparing for surgery. By working with weights and maintaining good nutrition, you can effectively build muscle. Push-ups, pull-ups, sit-ups, tai chi, and yoga exercises can also be used to build various muscle groups. Also, as we mentioned earlier, intensive, aerobic exercise boosts the body's production of growth hormone. This, in turn, stimulates protein synthesis in the muscle, thus accelerating the growth of new muscle.[16] Your level of aerobic fitness determines the effectiveness of your circulatory system and consequently your body's ability to deliver oxygen and nutrients. Therefore, getting into your best possible shape before surgery is critical to quick healing.

The ideal combination of exercise, then, involves resistance training coupled with aerobic exercise, such as running, swimming, or other vigorous athletic activities. This balance of muscle work and aerobic training enables you to establish whole-body fitness. It enables you to optimize aerobic fitness, while also improving muscle tone, flexibility, balance, and strength. Remember, too, that exercise not only strengthens the body, but also helps reduce stress and improves mood and attitude.

If you've been out of shape for some time, or if you've forgotten how to exercise well, you may want to check with your physician about a safe program for you. A personal fitness trainer can be an excellent guide. Through careful attention to your specific needs, a trainer can help launch you on your journey back to fitness and vitality. In some clinics, the physical therapist or exercise physiologist serves a similar role, though their training is more strongly grounded in the rehabilitation aspects of exercise and body-centered therapy.

Tending to Your Emotional Body

Preparing mentally for the challenge of surgery is also very useful. You can learn to calm your body and encourage deep relaxation through the use of guided imagery, deep breathing, and other relaxation techniques. Numerous studies have demonstrated the profound impact of these mind-body practices on clinical outcomes for people undergoing surgery. A simple relaxation script, for example, can greatly reduce the cost of your medical care because of the faster recovery that has been linked with such mind-body techniques in clinical studies.

In the next chapter, we walk you through some of the mind-body techniques we have found helpful in preparing our patients for surgery. How much stress and anxiety you experience just before the surgery can take away from your ability to heal afterward.[17] Patients who practice the various stress reduction techniques experience better energy levels, less postoperative pain and discomfort, less nausea, stronger immunity, fewer infections and other complications, and significantly faster recovery overall.[18]

Tending to Your Energetic Body

Your Energetic Body refers to a subtle form of energy that permeates the body and exerts a profound influence on your health. Five thousand years ago, Chinese medical doctors referred to this life force as Qi (pronounced "chee"), and stated that the flow and balance of this subtle energy was necessary for maintaining health. They used acupuncture, acupressure, herbs, and other methods to redress imbalances in the Qi. Of these approaches, acupuncture is the most prominent therapy to promote Qi flow along the meridians (energetic channels in the body).

Many studies have looked into the use of acupuncture before, during, and after surgery. A variety of techniques have been used, including traditional acupuncture (using needles), acupressure (applying manual pressure to acupoints), and electrostimulation of acupressure points. Acupuncture can aid in the prevention and treatment of nausea and pain during and shortly after surgery.[19] Acupuncture has also been shown to decrease the need for medications, shorten recovery time, and improve quality of recovery.[20] Many anesthesia departments now have licensed acupuncturists on staff or are willing to work with an acupuncturist.

Some of our patients came to hear about the benefits of acupuncture as the result of a remarkable study conducted by Dr. Tong Joo Gan and his anesthesiology colleagues at the Duke University Medical Center, which is located just down the road from our clinic. The study involved 40 women who were undergoing major breast surgery—either breast augmentation, breast reduction, or mastectomy—and requiring general anesthesia. The women were equally divided into three groups: one received acupuncture before the surgery, one received ondansetron (an antinausea drug better known as Zofran) prior to surgery, and one received a placebo pill. The researchers found that acupuncture proved better than the placebo and even better than traditional medications in reducing pain and nausea.[21] They found that the incidence and severity of nausea for acupuncture-treated patients was twice as low as the group receiving antinausea medication and four times lower than the group receiving the placebo.

Another controlled clinical trial, this one conducted in Japan, focused on the effects of acupuncture along the bladder meridian in patients scheduled for elective upper and lower abdominal surgery.[22] Before anesthesia, patients undergoing each type of surgery were randomly assigned to either acupuncture or the control group, which received sham or mock acupuncture. Starting from the recovery room, acupuncture significantly increased the number of patients who reported feeling good pain relief. And the acupuncture group also had 20 to 30 percent less postoperative nausea and 50 percent less need for morphine compared to the "fake acupuncture" group. At the same time, blood levels of the stress hormones cortisol and adrenaline (epinephrine) were reduced 30 to 50 percent in the acupuncture group during recovery and on the first day after the operation.

Acupressure is the "soft" counterpart to acupuncture. While acupuncture involves placing needles in energetic points, acupressure uses pressure from the practitioner's hands to press or massage these points to restore the balance of energy. Firm pressure on specific points along the meridians can promote energy flow to a part of the body that is experiencing pain or disease, and this in turn promotes healing and health. Using acupressure before surgery can also help prevent nausea and vomiting immediately after surgery. You can learn to apply acupressure to your own antinausea points before surgery—a routine and directions for specific points will be covered in chapter 6.

If this approach appeals to you, you may want to begin acupuncture in the weeks leading up to surgery. This will help you get used to the technique used, so that you'll have a greater level of comfort with acupuncture if you choose to have it *after* the surgery as well.

What follows is a massage routine you can do for yourself in the weeks before and after surgery to support general health, energy, and well-being. Place your fingertips in the center of your lower abdominal area, in the midline of the body between your belly button and pubic bone. Gradually press one to two inches deep inside the lower abdomen, 1½ inches below the belly button. This is called the *Sea of Energy* point (CV6). Rub gently in a circular motion for 1 to 2 minutes. Close your eyes as you breathe deeply.

Next, place your right heel on the outside of your left shinbone four finger widths below the knee, press in, then briskly rub the point up and down. This is called the *Three Mile* point (ST 36). After 1 minute, do the same on the other side.

You'll finish with the *Sea of Tranquility* (CV 17) point. With palms together, place the back of your thumbs firmly against the center of the breastbone at the level of your heart, three thumb widths up from the base of the bone. Continue to keep your eyes closed and concentrate on breathing slow, even, deep breaths into your heart to dispel any anxiety.

This little routine can be done sitting at a desk in 5 minutes. Be sure to keep the following guidelines in mind when doing acupressure. Never press on an open wound or acutely injured area or near a tumor. Certain points should not be used during pregnancy. Be sure to tell your practitioner if you are pregnant.

Another technique for strengthening your body's energy system is qigong (pronounced "chee-gong"). This ancient exercise practice from China is a regimen of focused breathing and movements that cultivate inner peace, balance, and greater energy. Regular daily practice can be enormously helpful to your healing.

❧ The Bottom Line: Preparing for Rapid Repair

If you're having an elective surgery, you should become as healthy as possible beforehand. You owe it to yourself to fortify your body for the physical and psychological challenges posed by the operation itself: the intense inflammation, oxidative stress, immune dysfunction, and other facets of the body's response to surgery.

Rarely do people begin taking concrete steps before surgery to ensure a more successful outcome. In this chapter, we've explained multiple ways you can prepare for this event. At the nutritional level, the strategies we recommend can help shift your body toward a biochemistry that is more conducive to optimal healing. At the physical or body-centered level, we urge you to consider getting in better shape and cutting out bad habits such as smoking. At the mind-body level, simply getting a better handle on your stress can help create the physiology to pave the way for a more favorable outcome. Energetically, acupuncture may be useful and can work synergistically with the other approaches.

The four levels of preparation—nutritional, physical, psychological, and energetic—are all mutually enhancing: by strengthening the body and building up key nutrient reserves, the mind strategies become more effective. By attending to the mind, the nutritional and physical care strategies become more effective.

In Table 4.4, we present the basic outline for a presurgery evaluation that could be helpful in determining how fit you are for surgery. If you have questions about how to interpret the table, be sure to consult with your doctor or surgical team. The first part of the table, which focuses on health habits and support, is common sense and should require no explanation. Nonetheless, it's important to keep the *overall balance* of factors in mind. For example, people who regularly engage in activities like gardening, swimming, tennis, riding a bike, jogging, golf (without a cart), or dancing obviously are more likely to be healthier, but if their dietary habits are bad or their daily stress levels too high, they may be less fit than you'd think. As you can see, the presurgery evaluation gives you the opportunity not only to modify your risk, but also to address key health issues that can have both short- and long-range consequences.

Where you may need professional guidance is in the second and third parts of the table, "Laboratory Tests" and "Clinical Observations," respectively. Keep in mind that the incidence of postsurgery complications is the highest in the first 48 hours after surgery (see chapter 6 for more details on these complications and how to prevent or manage them). Once you've moved past that point, you can breathe easier, but it's still important to be vigilant if you show some of the high-risk indicators in the first column, especially if you're older than age sixty-five or in poor overall health. (*Note:* We've tried to be as comprehensive as possible, but your physician may identify other potential areas of concern for your particular situation. For example, certain medications also should be evaluated before surgery. Aspirin and blood-thinning supplements should be discontinued at least one week before surgery. If you're taking an anticoagulant drug, you should discontinue it before surgery or switch to heparin at the time of surgery. Other medications that will require attention include diabetic medication, bronchodilator therapy, and steroids medication. Sedatives and certain other drugs may need to be tapered beforehand to prevent withdrawal reactions.)

In some instances, such as lower-back pain, you may elect to postpone surgery while exploring other options. In the case of lower-back pain due to a herniated disk, for example, you have a number of treatment options, such as a discectomy (removal of part of the leaking disk), a laminectomy (surgery to free up a pinched nerve), or spinal fusion, where the vertebrae are fused together. Or you may choose to have no surgery at all, relying instead on a combination of watchful waiting and natural methods—herbs, acupuncture, and mind-body techniques—to help you overcome the pain.

Part of the pre-op assessment, then, involves talking with your physician to decide whether to have surgery in the first place, based on a careful consideration of outcomes that are most important to you in the short and long terms. This kind of cautionary thinking helped shift medicine away from the once-routine practice of removing the tonsils. Two decades ago, tonsillectomies were commonplace, affecting about a million people a year—but then studies showed that in most cases the tonsils didn't need to be removed. Myringotomies, or insertion of tiny

Table 4.4. Pre-Op Assessment: Are You Fit for Surgery?

Indicators of Risk	Clinical Implications	Possible Course of Action*
I. Health Habits and Support		
Health-negating lifestyle: poor diet, physical inactivity, excessive psychological stress	Slower wound healing and increased risk of complications (e.g., high omega-6 and sugar intake may lead to increased inflammation)	Improve your nutrition by following the suggestions in chapters 3, 4, and 7. Get regular exercise, and get a handle on your stress (see chapter 5).
Substance abuse: smoking, drinking hard alcohol, and drug use	Increased risk of various surgical complications, nutritional problems, and delayed wound healing	Stop smoking or other substance abuse habits 4 to 8 weeks before surgery.
Poor social support	Slower wound healing and increased risk of complications due to emotional distress	Seek out friends and family for support; people who lack such support may require home services or temporary placement in a rehab facility post-surgery.
II. Laboratory Tests		
Albumin level less than 3.5 mg/dL (35 g/L). The normal range: (normal 3.5–5 mg/dL)	Increased risk of malnutrition, infections, and other postsurgery complications; potentially delayed wound healing	Increase intake of protein and calories (from good fat and carbohydrate sources); if malnutrition is severe, consider postponing surgery and providing preoperative supplementation.

Lymphocyte count less than 1,500 cells/mm3	Increased risk of malnutrition, delayed wound healing, and post-surgery complications	Improve immune system competence through diet, exercise, and stress management; consult with a holistic immunologist.
High blood sugar levels: fasting plasma glucose higher than 100 mg/dL, especially for someone older than forty-five years or with a history of diabetes	Increased risk of delayed wound healing and postsurgery complications	Take steps to improve your blood sugar control, see dietary suggestions in chapter 4 and supplement suggestions for diabetics or borderline diabetics in chapter 8.
Urinalysis and liver function tests with abnormal results	Increased risk for kidney or liver problems after surgery	Medications and anesthesia levels will need to be adjusted; urinary tract infections should be treated before surgery.

III. Clinical Observations

Obesity: BMI of 30 or more (ideal BMI is 19 to 25, though percent body fat or skinfold thickness should also be considered in very muscular individuals)	Increased risk of complications and delayed healing	Postpone procedure until body composition has been improved (reduced body fat, increased muscle); take additional measures to reduce inflammatory potential well before surgery (e.g., omega-3 supplements).

High blood pressure, heart murmurs, unstable angina, signs of congestive heart failure, myocardial infarction within six weeks, and aortic or peripheral vascular surgery	Increased risk for cardiac and cardiopulmonary complications (e.g., ischemia) during and after the surgery Patients at highest risk: those who face emergency surgery, those with anticipated increased blood loss, and those having aortic or peripheral vascular surgery; patients at intermediate risk: those receiving abdominal or thoracic surgery, head and neck surgery, carotid endarterectomy, orthopedic or prostate surgery	Postpone procedure until cardiac indicators or cardiac stress testing results are more favorable; the type of surgery influences overall risk and the need for further cardiac evaluation and careful monitoring—an ECG should be obtained in people older than forty years or in those with cardiac indications based on the past medical history; consult with a cardiologist before having surgery.
Respiratory disease such as asthma, obstructive pulmonary disease, shortness of breath (dyspnea)	Increased risk of pulmonary complications during and after surgery	Postpone procedure until pulmonary indicators are more stable or favorable; pulmonary function tests and a chest X-ray may be used to assess fitness for surgery; some patients may benefit from perioperative use of bronchodilators or steroids and should receive instruction in deep-breathing exercises or incentive spirometry; pulmonary function testing or peak flow rate to assess disease status; consult with a pulmonary specialist (lung doctor) before having surgery.

High risk for bleeding due to type of procedure	Increased risk for transfusion	Will need to have a blood-typing test done; may want to consider banking own blood.
Persistent fever, wheezing, or significant nasal discharge	Increased risk of respiratory tract infection during and after surgery	Antimicrobial treatment may be needed or surgery may need to be postponed; consult with an infectious-disease specialist before having surgery.

*These options should, of course, be discussed with your physician.

Note: Other tests may also be considered for specific circumstances. Consider a urine pregnancy test if you're a woman of childbearing age. Coagulation tests are needed if you're receiving anticoagulant therapy, have a family or personal history that suggests a bleeding disorder, or have evidence of liver disease. Measurement of your hemoglobin level can indicate the presence of anemia and also provides baseline information that can be helpful postsurgery, particularly for surgeries with potential hemorrhagic complications.

tubes to prevent recurrent ear infection (usually in children), is another one of those overused surgical procedures that may soon go the way of tonsillectomies. Gallbladder removal, cataract surgery, hysterectomy, cesarean section (C-section), prostatectomy (for early stage, low-grade prostate cancer), and surgeries for jaw pain and sleep apnea are other examples of procedures that might warrant a second or third opinion before you give your surgeon the green light.

Now that we've provided you with the guidance you need to get your body-mind organism in tip-top condition, let's look at steps you can take to cope more effectively with the experience of the surgery. Some of these steps can be taken in the 2 days prior to surgery, as well as on the day of the actual operation. Even within the operating room, there are things you can do to help you recover more quickly.

5

Using Your Inner Healer During Your Operation

*Peace is always there, to some extent.
And if you know how to practice
[mindfulness], then you can always be
in touch with peace, to some degree, for
your nourishment and healing.*

—THICH NHAT HANH

Beth Ann had given birth to her fifth child, a beautiful boy with deep brown eyes and jet-black hair. She was intent on this being her last birth, but had had the same intention when her fourth child was born. The diaphragm had been hard to remember, her IUD had fallen out, and pills had made her too moody. She did not want to take any more chances. Her partner kept putting off the vasectomy, and she wanted to do something soon. Although she knew she did not want any more children, she also regarded surgery with some trepidation—it just seemed too radical a solution.

After explaining what to expect on the physical level from a laparoscopy, I could sense that the fear went deeper than the surgery itself. My experience with other women facing similar circumstances had taught me that surgeries to the pelvis often have a profound emotional resonance. The pelvic organs relate to sexuality, femininity (or masculinity), creativity, and a sense of personal power. I wondered if ligating her tubes in some way symbolized for her a cutting off of one of these essential functions. I suggested to her that many people feel more creative or sexually free when the fear of pregnancy is removed, and I asked her to try journaling or drawing an image about the surgery to help her access her fears and better work through them.

When Beth Ann returned for her pre-op visit, she told me she had drawn a cage. When I asked about the cage and its meaning, she related it to an episode of date rape she'd experienced in college. After several years of therapy, she had managed to put the experience behind her, but the idea of being powerless under anesthesia while her tubes where cut brought the issue back to the surface again.

It seemed clear to me that Beth Ann needed to be in control of her body and the situation. Most women who have this procedure do so under general anesthesia. In Beth Ann's case, however, I felt she might feel more secure if she was awake and could talk to me. She agreed with me on this point. I then suggested relaxation breathing, hypnosis, and acupuncture as adjuncts to local anesthesia so that she could be awake and in control during the entire procedure. I gave her some mini-breathing exercises to practice at home whenever she started to think or feel anxious about the procedure.

Lastly, I suggested a visualization to practice that involved transforming the cage in her mind to a beautiful creative space with wide open doors and windows with a beautiful view. With five children, Beth Ann did not have much time to practice, but she was able to use the guided visualization for a few minutes in the bath or shower each day in the two weeks before surgery.

During the procedure she continued to use these techniques. I talked her through the procedure as she watched on the monitor. Her ability to control the situation with breathing and letting go of negative thoughts helped the entire procedure go more easily. She left the OR feeling calm, happy, and more empowered then ever.

—EGM

Imagine facing surgery 6,000 years ago, when the Egyptians and Peruvians performed the first operations in recorded history. The instruments for making incisions were no doubt very crude, a far cry from the sleek, stainless-steel scalpels used by today's surgeons. And, of course, this was long before the advent of sterilization and pain-killing pharmaceuticals. The risks to the patient would have been substantial. The first effective forms of anesthesia—ether, nitrous oxide ("laughing gas"), and chloroform—came into use much later, all three being introduced in the 1840s.[1] Although ancient physicians did use natural methods such as herbs and acupuncture to help manage pain, people undergoing surgery in ancient times had to rely a great deal on their inner resources, on the mind's capacities for promoting profound relaxation and inner peace.

Major surgery puts your body through a tremendous amount of stress. Like it or not, when you submit to going "under the knife," your body unleashes a virtual tsunami of stress chemicals such as cortisol and catecholamines. These so-called fight-or-flight hormones tend to weaken your immune system and increase the breakdown of muscle and other tissues. When these stress chemicals remain elevated for an extended period of time, your nutritional reserves are more readily depleted, and this, in turn, tends to diminish your body's wound-healing abilities.

As if this isn't enough, there's also the emotional distress that comes with facing major surgery. Anxiety, fatigue, and depression can add to the stress-hormone chemistry that's triggered by the surgery itself. Learning to cope with your fears about surgery is an important way to reduce stress. These fears are entirely justified. Because of surgery, you may experience pain, disability, and loss of organs or organ function. You may have to deal with the effects of being away from home and family and a loss of the ability to be productive, but the amount of suffering you encounter from these changes can be minimized if you have access to the mind-body techniques described in this chapter. With counseling, support, and relaxation techniques you'll be much better able to handle both the emotional and physical stresses of surgery.

A 2003 report from the University of Auckland in New Zealand helps illustrate just how powerful the stress connection really is.[2] The study focused on 47 adults who were being operated on for severe hernia. Each participant was given a standardized questionnaire to assess psychological stress–and in particular, the level of worry concerning the operation. In the first 20 hours after the surgery, the researchers collected and then analyzed fluid from the surgical wound. Intriguingly, the greater the degree of perceived stress, the lower the levels of various substances known to be involved in wound healing. The researchers concluded that "psychological stress impairs the inflammatory response and is antithetical to healing."

The collective effects of stress explain why an integrative approach to surgery makes the most sense: bringing together specific forms of nutritional support that can help counteract the "chemistry of stress," while using mind-body practices to further bolster your internal resilience and exploit your full self-healing potential.

In chapter 4, we focused on the nutritional side of the equation. Here we will focus on what you can accomplish using your "inner healer," your mind and consciousness, or what might be called your emotional body. By directing the mind in a positive way toward the experience of surgery and its aftermath, you will take full advantage of your body's healing capacities, and your recovery will be less stressful and more efficient. Many studies have shown that whereas psychological stress delays the healing of wounds, relaxation and inner harmony tend to strengthen and accelerate the healing process.[3]

Of course, stress is not a one-way street but depends to a very large degree on how your mind perceives and responds to the challenge of surgery. Your "mind's eye" is just as important in coping with pain as drugs and medical procedures—and how you direct your consciousness around the time of surgery can yield far more powerful outcomes than we usually give credit for. By learning to deeply relax yourself and to connect with what you are feeling at a given moment, your surgical experience will be more positive, and you're far more likely to recuperate faster and more harmoniously after the operation.

Specifically, the mind-body techniques we will describe can help you achieve the following five objectives:

- A calmer, more relaxed state of being before the operation and, in particular, just as you are about to undergo surgery
- Less pain after surgery, and therefore a reduced need for pain medications

- A stronger immune system, resulting in a lower risk of infection
- A reduced risk of complications, garnering you considerable savings on medical bills
- Enhanced tissue repair and thus a more rapid recovery

Your ability to harness the healing forces within you is virtually unlimited. Even so, a certain amount of practice can help you tap into these forces more effectively in times of stress and tension. If you have never used relaxation techniques in the past, we would encourage you to begin practicing one or more of these as soon as possible, ideally several weeks before the operation. But even if you have only a few days to prepare for the operation, this chapter can come in very handy.

✖ Different Roads to the Inner Landscape

The art of mind-body medicine recognizes that there are many different ways to achieve internal resilience, relaxation, and peace of mind. In this chapter, we introduce you to just a few of the methods we believe are most effective in the context of preparing for surgery.

Your mind and your body are linked through a two-way communications system we call the central nervous system. Mind and body not only *can* communicate with each other, they probably do so all the time at a level far beyond our conscious awareness. How does this occur? At one level, we have the wiring of nerves that permeate most of our tissues, glands, and organs. But we also have a number of nerve chemicals, called neuropeptides, which mediate our emotions. As neurobiologist Candace Pert teaches us, the receptors for neuropeptides are found in almost every cell in the body, which may explain, in part, why emotions can affect so many different parts of the body.[4]

Harvard cardiologist Herbert Benson was among the first scientists to probe the profound healing connection between the mind and body. In the early 1970s, Dr. Benson demonstrated that training people in various relaxation techniques led to beneficial changes in the body, all of which amounted to what he termed the *relaxation response*.[5] The main changes included slower breathing, reduced heart rate, reduced use of oxygen, and lower levels of a metabolic toxin called lac-

—Stress Strikes at the Genetic Level—

Stress is profoundly linked to healing and aging, not just in terms of our outward appearance, but also at the cellular level and even at the molecular level. As we get older, our genetic material gradually loses its stability. One symptom of this decline is a shortening of our telomeres, the tips or ends of the chromosomes that carry our genes. Telomeres are required for DNA replication and stability, and there now appears to be a strong connection between how fast we age and the shortening of our telomeres.[6] Apparently, the telomeres eventually get so short that cells can no longer divide, and they die prematurely—hence premature aging.

Telomeres are also linked with our capacity for wound healing.[7] Animal studies show that the shortening of telomeres with age is accompanied by a shortened life span *and* a reduced capacity for wound healing.[8] This makes sense, given that wound healing is a process that entails the formation of new tissues, hence plenty of DNA replication. It also helps explain why elderly people, who tend to have shorter telomeres, show a diminished capacity for tissue repair or healing.

Until recently, telomere attrition in humans was thought to be due mainly to free radicals and chronic inflammation (and not surprisingly, by the way, a number of antioxidants may help curb telomere losses).[9] We now know that psychological stress also plays a role. Researchers at the University of California, San Francisco studied women aged twenty to fifty who had been stressed by caring for a child with a serious chronic illness. The telomeres of these women were then compared to those of women with healthy children (the low-stress or control group). The women in the high-stress group showed the greatest deterioration of their telomeres: their telomeres were shorter on average by about a decade compared to women in the low-stress group.[10]

tic acid. Since Benson's original research, the relaxation response has emerged as a therapeutic tool that can counteract a variety of cardiovascular, immune, and neurodegenerative disorders.[11]

Many different exercises can elicit the relaxation response. These include progressive muscle relaxation, guided imagery, hypnosis, meditation, and various breathing exercises. Progressive muscle relaxation involves consciously and gradually releasing each muscle group in the body. Guided imagery entails use of the imagination or a taped sequence to conjure peaceful images in the mind, such as a beach, mountain scene, or favorite place, to take the mind off fearful thoughts. Anxiety is replaced by the sound of the ocean, the feel of the breeze. Positive affirmations, hypnosis, and self-hypnosis are techniques that focus the mind on helpful suggestions such as "your body knows how to heal completely and easily." Meditation can also be used to take the mind off fearful and negative thoughts. The meditator focuses the mind on the breath or a mantra (a special word like peace or healing). The slow, deep breathing that accompanies most of these techniques is also in itself relaxing. Each of these methods will be explained further in this chapter.

With a little practice, you will find that all of these techniques are relatively easy to learn. They have been shown to be very helpful in many medical situations, providing relief for high blood pressure, pain (both acute and chronic), insomnia, headache, irritable bowel syndrome, infertility, and coronary artery disease.[12] And, of course, they've also been shown to help in preparing for and recovering from surgery.

All of the techniques that elicit the relaxation response can be looked at as different forms of *self-regulation*. In other words, they are designed to give you a greater sense of control, to make you more at home with your own mind. They can also help you accomplish certain life-enhancing goals. For example, if you feel tension creeping up into your shoulders, there are soothing images, self-statements, and breathing techniques you can use to release this tension before it becomes chronic, burdensome, or even disabling. The more you practice these self-regulation strategies, the more inner peace and stability you're likely to experience over time.

✎ Self-Regulation Strategies before and after Surgery

The four stress-reducing strategies we teach to people for use before and after surgery are the following: (1) *hypnosis* (including self-hypnosis), coupled with either relaxation imagery or healing self-statements, (2) *mindful breathing,* (3) *calming music,* and (4) *soothing statements* your own surgeon or anesthesiologist can articulate during your operation, for added support. Additionally, the use of a support group and "healing team" is worth exploring, as we will discuss toward the end of the chapter. These methods can further strengthen you for the surgery—in ways entirely complementary to nutrition and body-centered care—and get your body in tip-top healing condition.

Let's now take a look at some of the methods we have found most helpful in the context of surgery, beginning with hypnosis.

✎ Training the Mind for Rapid Repair: The Power of Trance

For thousands of years, people have used hypnosis, or trance work, for healing purposes. Psychologists today use it primarily to help people resolve emotional traumas, change long-standing habits, and improve performance. In the context of surgery, better pain management is perhaps the best-studied effect of hypnosis. A preoperative hypnosis session can also markedly reduce your need for analgesic drugs after the operation.[13] Moreover, there are many documented examples of people going through major surgery with self-hypnosis as their sole form of anesthesia.[14] This particular application, called *hypnoanesthesia,* is a potential life saver for individuals who have a bad reaction to real anesthesia, or for people in third world and developing countries, where anesthesia is unavailable or at least hard to come by.

What exactly is hypnosis? Hypnosis can be defined as a state of heightened awareness and focused concentration. In this sense it is similar to meditation. But whereas meditation is classically defined as a practice that cultivates present-moment awareness, hypnosis is more goal oriented and can be used for multiple purposes. In addition to being used to transform your perception of pain, it has also been effective in curbing anxiety and nausea before an operation, limiting blood loss, speeding up tissue repair, and shortening hospital stays.[15] The hypnotic state, also known as *trance,* is a relaxing, naturally occurring state of mind that happens to all of us at one time or another. Whenever you become completely engrossed in a novel or movie, or whenever you allow yourself to float off in a daydream—transporting yourself to another time and place—you're experiencing at least a mild trance.

Hypnosis is very effective when combined with a guided imagery sequence. For example, you might be asked to focus on a favorite memory. Images of natural scenery or a favorite childhood memory are often conjured up for this purpose. By fully concentrating on pleasant, soothing imagery during surgery, you can enter into a sublimely peaceful state. Whether you're using hypnosis or self-hypnosis, the fundamental goal is to get your unconscious mind to *communicate with your body.* This is done by first bringing the body into a state of deep relaxation or trance. Once there, your "unconscious" and thus your entire body may become receptive to hypnotic suggestions. When you listen to these suggestions, either uttered by an experienced hypnotist or as part of an audio recording to which you can listen just before going into surgery, your body-mind will be receptive and ready to absorb them as fully as possible. Here are two examples of hypnotic suggestions that can be given before surgery, once you've entered into the state of deep relaxation (see page 105 for additional examples):

"When you wake up from your operation, you will feel healthier and more refreshed than ever before."

"When you wake up, you will feel energized, refreshed, and free of all pain."

You may use a variety of other statements after the operation to reinforce the healing process—statements that can be made either by yourself or by a friend or loved one. (At the end of this section, we provide some resources for finding additional examples of hypnosis statements and scripts for a variety of situations.) Here are two:

"Your skin is mending rapidly, becoming smooth and resilient."

"Your tissues are knitting together rapidly, becoming stronger each day as you continue to nourish your body with healing foods and nutrients."

As for how hypnosis actually influences the healing process, this is still being studied. What we do know is that hypnosis can favorably affect the inflammatory response, activate key regions of the brain, and bolster your immune system. And the bottom line is that it works quite well for people facing surgery and recovering from surgery, as demonstrated in a controlled study of women receiving *mammaplasty,* a reconstruction of the breast to reduce size and weight of mammary tissue.[16] The researchers, led by psychologist Carol Ginandes of Harvard Medical School, chose three groups for comparison. The first was a support group in which people were encouraged to simply express their feelings about the surgery. The second group included people who received only the usual care, such as follow-up doctor visits. These two groups were then compared with women who received hypnosis before and after surgery.

Women in the hypnosis group received eight half-hour sessions per week for 2 weeks before surgery, and then for 6 weeks afterward. All of these sessions involved the use of a scripted set of hypnotic statements. The suggestions were aimed at a smooth surgery experience, reduced bleeding at the surgical site, a decrease in painful sensations, and expectations for rapid healing after the operation. None of the medical staff that measured the healing of wounds after surgery knew which women were in the hypnosis groups—they were "blinded" in order to avoid biasing the results.

Here's what Dr. Ginandes found: the hypnosis sessions led to a statistically significant increase in the rate of wound healing compared to the other two groups. After both 1 week and then again 7 weeks following the operation, the hypnosis group was showing better scores on postoperative pain, overall functioning, and healing of their incisions.

Most other hypnosis research has focused primarily on the management of postoperative pain. In a 3-year study by surgeons at the University of Liege in Belgium, patients undergoing various thyroid-related surgeries were assigned to one of two groups.[17] Ninety percent of these surgeries involved removal of the thyroid gland, while the rest were exploratory neck operations. One group of patients received *hypnosedation,* meaning that they went without regular anesthesia and were guided into a state of deep relaxation before being operated on. These patients were then compared to a similar ("matched") population of patients undergoing the same types of surgery, but with general anesthesia instead of hypnosedation. Here's what the Belgian study showed.

- All the surgeons reported better operating conditions (for example, more stable heart rate) for the patients who had undergone hypnosedation.

- Only 1 percent of the hypnotized patients had to be switched over to general anesthesia during the operation.

- All patients in the hypnosis group reported having had a "very pleasant experience" during surgery, according to the researchers.

- Hypnotized patients also experienced significantly less postoperative pain and required fewer pain-killing medications than the other two groups.

- The hospital stay was significantly shorter for patients in the hypnosis group, resulting in a substantial reduction in medical care bills.

- Patients who had undergone hypnosedation returned to their social or professional activities significantly sooner than those in the general anesthesia group.

As you can see, hypnosis seems to be a very efficient way to provide physical, psychological, and economic benefits to people undergoing surgery. Other studies have revealed similarly strong outcomes. In a study at the Southeastern Louisiana University School of Nursing, men and women undergoing gallbladder surgery (cholecystectomy) were randomly assigned to either deep relaxation with guided imagery or a simple quiet period before going into surgery.[18] After the operation, patients who had practiced the guided imagery showed significantly less anxiety, lower stress hormone levels following surgery, and less inflammation (erythema) around the wound area than the ones who had the quiet period. All of these stress-relieving outcomes have been linked with better healing.

There are many books and Web sites (e.g., www.hypnosis.com and www.hypnosis-japan.org/scriptlinks.html) where you can find examples of hypnotic healing suggestions. After you've read some examples, feel free to create suggestions that apply to your individual situation and needs. Many psychologists are trained in hypnosis—check your yellow pages under hypnotherapy if you'd feel more comfortable working with a licensed provider.

Healing Statements During the Surgery

In addition to the benefits of hypnosis or trance work before and after surgery, there's also evidence that such mind states can be beneficial when people are actually undergoing surgery as well.

In a study published in the British medical journal *Lancet,* psychiatrist Carleton Evans and his colleagues at Guy's Hospital in London offered therapeutic suggestions to 39 women under general anesthesia for their hysterectomies.[19] The surgical team played a tape for half the women *during* the surgery. The recorded statements were designed to help the women relax and feel more confident about the surgery. None of the women in the study knew beforehand—that is, before "going under"—whether they were going to have the soothing statements read during the surgery. Women who received the positive suggestions recovered more quickly from the operation. They also suffered fewer complications and spent significantly less time in the hospital after the surgery.

As you can see, hypnosis can be very useful for surgical patients. Keep in mind, though, that you need to be motivated in order to benefit from hypnosis or self-hypnosis. This is not a passive experience, nor is it a given that hypnosis is going to work for you. Some people are more open to hypnotic suggestion than others. This has nothing to do with gullibility, only with different levels of receptivity. A well-trained psychologist will be able to determine how suggestible you are. Many people can learn to be hypnotized and, for some, it's just a matter of finding the right technique. Again, we'd recommend that you take a look at the various books and Web sites (e.g., www.hypnosis.com) for additional insights on how to use this powerful mind-body technique.

❧ Mindful Breathing

One of the best ways you can keep your mind firmly planted in the present moment is by paying impartial attention to the rhythmic movement of your own breath. Dr. Herbert Benson's basic technique for inducing relaxation, in fact, involved the mindful coordinating of in-breath and out-breath–simply observing the ebb and flow of the breath. If a distracting thought or emotion arises, the person practices letting go in a nonjudging way and returns to gently watching the

—The Ginandes Approach for People Facing Surgery—

Dr. Carol Ginandes, a Harvard-affiliated health psychologist, integrates medical hypnosis into her work with patients coming to her for mind-body support. She has done collaborative research with Dr. Dan Rosenthal and Dr. Patricia Brooks, showing that hypnosis can be used to accelerate healing of bone fractures as well as tissue healing following surgery.[20]

In her clinical work, Dr. Ginandes creates comprehensive guided visualization interventions, offered in multiple sessions as an adjunct to standard medical care. Her approach provides a sequence of guided self-hypnotic exercises that have been designed to help patients navigate the different tasks and phases of healing from injury, illness, or surgery.

By utilizing a carefully interwoven set of suggestions, the patient first learns to access a self-hypnotic state of *inner absorption at will*. Once this has been mastered with practice, suggestions for comfort and calm can help to alleviate preoperative anxieties and to anticipate a smooth procedure.

After surgery, patients learn how to use vivid inner imagery to cultivate the return of normal bodily functioning, diminish pain, soothe inflammation, rebuild healthy tissue, and recover vitality over the course of days and weeks. Dr. Ginandes emphasizes that emotional concerns about the procedure or injury are important to address as well. Rehabilitative tasks include the return of strength, functionality, and flexibility over the course of weeks after surgery or injury.[21]

The extensive transcripts of these interventions, which use a complex series of targeted suggestions over multiple sessions, are beyond the scope of this chapter. Nonetheless, these very useful audio programs for recovery from surgery and injury are available at this Web site (www.healthjourneys.com) or by contacting Dr. Ginandes directly.[22]

We present some of the suggestions used in the Ginandes audio programs series below. Each suggestion has been extracted from its original context and is cited only for the purpose of illustration. Dr. Ginandes emphasizes that the suggestions are not meant to be used independently of her full hypnosis protocol.

Some Preoperative Suggestions

- As you prepare to go through surgery, learn how to take an inner vacation to a healing sanctuary where you will have all the comfort you need.
- It's natural to have some anxiety before a procedure. But you can cultivate a feeling of peace, comfort, and relaxation. Since you are not helpless, you can use your mind to modify your body's responses and to help it go through the procedure and heal quickly and well.
- You can even help your body bleed very little during surgery by constricting the tiny little blood vessels and by shunting the blood away from the operative site to other parts of your body during the procedure.

Some Postoperative Suggestions

- You can allow all of your bodily functions to make their way toward their normal state as you rest and replenish yourself.
- Soon you will feel thirsty and hungry and be looking forward to your next meal. The surgery has accomplished its purpose, and, from now on, your immune system can powerfully facilitate your healing rapidly and well.
- Of course, we all know that most surgeries are accompanied by pain; actually, pain is a very useful alarm system built into your body to alert you that something needs your attention. But once you have gotten medical attention for it, you don't want to have that alarm bell ringing again and again. There is no gain from that pain. By simply allowing that discomfort to recede as a ship disappears over the horizon right before your very eyes, a wave of comfort and relief can flow in.
- As you plan for your return home, remind yourself of the things that you are looking forward to, such as attending a particular event or just realizing that the surgery is behind you.
- As you get and remain more comfortable, your body can go about the business of healing your incisions rapidly

and well. In your mind's eye, try to see the area renewing itself, maybe using your powerful imagination to create a special imaginary healing cream to apply to the surgical site to soothe and speed the healing.

breath. This gentle, repetitive focus has a calming effect that, with practice, can lead to ever deeper states of relaxation. Some people find it helpful to count slowly on the inhale (1, 2, 3, etc.) before beginning the count again on the exhale. Others find it easier to imagine the air coming in as cleansing, and the air going out as carrying toxic energy. After a short while, your breathing pattern begins to resemble that of restful sleep.

Yogic breathing practices are widely used to help release tension in the body. Hatha yoga teaches us to take a few long, slow breaths, letting the air flow downward deeply into our lungs until it "feels" as though it has reached and permeated the entire abdomen, then afterward slowly exhaling the breath until the last air seeps out. The individual becomes more firmly "grounded" in the body by visualizing the flow of air downward through the body on the inhale and flowing out through the soles of the feet on the exhale.

Deep breathing exercises such as these, perhaps coupled with some simple yoga postures, such as standing forward bends, are usually effective ways to cope with an upsurge of anxiety. They can be used at any time, and require no technological or expert assistance. As such, they comprise an indispensable tool to help you relax before and after surgery.

Many hospitals and integrative medical clinics offer 8-week courses in mindfulness-based stress reduction. Check your local paper or the Internet for more information. There are many books and audiotapes available as well. Look for such materials by Jon Kabat-Zinn (www.mindfulnesstapes.com), a pioneer in this field as well as someone who continues to practice and offer seminars nationally. Another resource can be your local yoga studio—look for classes that focus on gentle stretching and relaxation, or what is increasingly referred to as "restorative yoga."

ᔇ Progressive Muscle Relaxation

Another method that has been used to help induce a state of deep relaxation and relieve pain is progressive muscular relaxation, or PMR. One of the most common signs of being "stressed out" is chronic muscular tension, which often manifests as painful tightness, hardness, or "knots" in the neck and shoulder muscles. PMR is a technique for releasing such tension and breaking the vicious cycle of pain, muscle constriction, and anxiety. Recent research suggests that it may be helpful in helping alleviate the stress and tension many patients experience around the time of surgery.[23]

The basic method of PMR is to tense up a group of muscles as strongly as possible and hold them in a state of extreme tension for a few seconds. You then allow the muscles to return to their previous state, and finally you consciously relax them as much as you can. For example, you can practice this technique by forming a fist and keeping it intensely clenched for a few seconds. Next, relax your hand to its previous tension, and then consciously allow it to become even more relaxed. With a little practice, this should result in a feeling of deep relaxation in your hands and forearms. The same basic technique can be applied to any or all of the muscle groups in your body; very often, you will feel an enormous sense of relief as the tension eases up in one area or another.

Dr. Carol Mandle and colleagues at Harvard Medical School studied patients who received training in PMR prior to a minor surgical procedure called angiography.[24] This procedure involves puncturing an artery (in this case, in the thigh area) in order to insert a catheter for diagnostic purposes. Forty-five angiography patients were given one of three types of audiotapes: a relaxation response tape with PMR, a tape of contemporary music, or a blank tape. All patients were instructed to listen to their audiotape, using headphones, during the entire procedure. The patients given the PMR audiotape experienced less anxiety, less pain, and required less pain medication during the procedure compared to patients given either the music or the blank audiotapes. This is consistent with many other studies showing a reduction in medication use for people who practice relaxation techniques.[25]

You may want to use PMR in conjunction with breathing techniques and imagery for optimal relaxation. Also, try starting with areas where you clearly sense the most tension—a clenched jaw, rock-hard shoulders, tension in your neck, or a knot in your stomach. Although this approach does not get rid of the emotional distress that may be creating the tension, it can enable you to function well and respond better to other mind-body strategies.

❧ During the Operation: Soothing Statements

We usually assume that we only hear and sense things when we're conscious, but this just isn't the case. There is overwhelming scientific evidence that you can perceive and encode meaningful information *even when you're unconscious,* as you would be under general anesthesia. In addition to receiving auditory stimuli, patients can also respond to verbal cues during an operation—for example, by tensing up their muscles.[26] In one study, patients were given various kinds of information while under anesthesia; after regaining consciousness, testing indicated that they had indeed retained much of this information.[27] Many patients can recall noises and comments that were made by the surgical team during the operation.[28]

There are certain therapeutic advantages to being able to perceive and record things that are said by your surgeon or by others in the operating room. In 1990, researchers in Glasgow, Scotland, studied 63 women having total abdominal hysterectomies.[29] During surgery, while under general anesthesia, half of this group received the following recorded suggestion: "You will feel warm and comfortable, calm and relaxed; any pain that you feel after the operation will not concern you." Patients who received the therapeutic suggestion reported experiencing less pain immediately after surgery and required significantly less morphine on the day of the operation than the control group.

Two years earlier, a similar study involving the same surgery had been conducted at St. Thomas' Hospital in London.[30] This time, however, the surgeons themselves voiced the following therapeutic suggestions during the operation: "How quickly you recover from your operation depends upon you—the more you relax, the more comfortable you will be. You will not feel sick; you will not have any pain. The operation seems to be going very well, and the patient is fine."

Women in the therapeutic suggestion group experienced significantly less fever symptoms (indicating less infection), spent less time in the hospital after surgery, and had a better overall recovery, according to their nurses.

As with the Glasgow study, this was a double-blind, placebo-controlled clinical trial, so that the health care providers who evaluated the outcomes did not know which patients had actually received the therapeutic suggestions. Other research has confirmed these findings.[31] For example, a study at New York University Medical Center showed that therapeutic suggestions offered under anesthesia resulted in the following postoperative benefits: less nausea, fewer headaches, and less muscular discomfort.[32]

At this writing, there are twice as many studies showing a favorable influence of healing statements offered during surgery as there are studies showing no benefit (a score of four to two). Our conclusion is that because it certainly can't hurt to receive such suggestions, it is worth approaching your surgeon in the following way:

- First, explain that you have read about some of the research on giving positive statements during surgery, and that you would appreciate having this additional support. Although your surgeon need not understand the mind-body connection, it's certainly helpful to have one who respects your personal needs. If this particular mind-body practice is important for you, and your surgeon is unwilling to cooperate, then you may want to ask the anesthesiologist instead. Having the anesthesiologist do it also works well.

- Second, ask your surgeon to verbalize the statements in Table 5.1 during the surgery. You may also ask that your surgeon and OR staff refrain from making "negative" statements about your condition while you are under anesthesia.

- Third, offer the four statements provided by Peggy Huddleston in her excellent book on mind-body techniques, *Prepare for Surgery, Heal Faster* (Cambridge, MA: Angel River Press, 1996). These statements are shown in Table 5.1.

Table 5.1. Four Healing Suggestions to Be Given During Surgery*

Statement	Huddleston's practical notes
1. "Following this operation, you will feel comfortable and you will heal very well."	This statement may help reduce pain and speed up healing after the operation. If you will be unconscious during the operation, this should be repeated five times as you are going under anesthesia. If you will be awake, it should be repeated five times while you are deeply relaxed (gentle deep breathing) at the beginning of the operation.
2. "Your operation has gone very well. I am very pleased with your_____." (Fill in the blank: hip, shoulder, etc.)	This statement may help you feel more relaxed or less stressed during the surgery, and again may accelerate your recovery. It should be repeated five times toward the end of surgery.
3. "Following this operation, you will wake up hungry for _____. You will be thirsty and you will be able to urinate easily." (Fill in the blank with the name of your favorite light, healthy food, such as pasta, soup, whole-grain toast, etc.)	This statement sends a signal to your digestive and elimination systems to return to normal functioning. This can help prevent the medical complications that may arise when these systems are sluggish due to anesthesia. The statement should be repeated five times toward the end of surgery.
4. "Following this operation, _____." (Fill in the blank with positive words your surgeon or primary physician recommends for your recovery.)	This statement should describe your healing process graphically, explaining something basic about the physiology of your recovery. You and your physician can draft it together. Examples include phrases like "your tissues will knit together quickly." Again, the statement should be repeated five times toward the end of surgery.

*Adapted from *Prepare for Surgery, Heal Faster: A Guide of Mind-Body Techniques,* by Peggy Huddleston (Cambridge, MA: Angel River Press, 1996), pp. 151–63.

Keep in mind that additional statements may be tailored for your particular situation. For example, with an operation that may involve extensive bleeding, Huddleston offers the following suggestion: "You'll have minimal bleeding during the surgery." (This is repeated five times as surgery begins.) As more research accumulates, these healing statements may become part of the surgeon's code of conduct in the operating room.

✌ During the Operation: Calming Music

Music can have a healing effect. We know this intuitively, as some forms of music seem to transport us to a place of profound solace and serenity. At the same time, noise or dissonance can be disturbing, stressful, irritating. There's some evidence that a noisy environment may prolong hospital stays.[33] And we know that the typical noise level in an operating room can be substantial, from the bleeping of monitors to the clanking of surgical instruments as they are dropped into metal pans to the conversations of surgical team members to the beeping of pagers and the occasional blaring of loud music on loudspeakers.

Given that auditory stimuli are picked up even when we're unconscious, such noise could have unwanted effects on a surgical outcome. At the same time, the opposite influence—soothing music—seems to be beneficial. To begin with, soothing music may help keep distracting noises and statements from causing distress and raising your heart rate. We know that patients who listen to their favorite music do show lower anxiety and stress hormone levels during surgery and experience less pain as well.[34] The use of "sedative music" during open-heart surgery results in a significant reduction in anxiety and pain after the operation when compared to scheduled rest or the usual treatment.[35]

Given the connections between stress and poor wound healing, one might expect that listening to a calming, melodious tune during your operation could help wound healing as well. At least one study found that either music, or music accompanied by therapeutic suggestions, resulted in a speedier recovery for patients who underwent hysterectomies.[36] Clearly, then, the use of music may be a simple, inexpensive, and easily used strategy for minimizing anxiety and pain, and for improving your overall experience of surgery and post-op recovery.

If you do opt for listening to music during surgery, listen to something with a background beat of about 60 to 80 beats/minute. Your heart rate will tend to synchronize with the beat you are listening to, and you want to maintain a calm and steady rate throughout the procedure. Check to see if your hospital has a CD or tape player in the OR. Otherwise, bring a portable player. Put your name and number on any music or players you bring to the hospital. Remember to replace old batteries beforehand and set the auto reverse on (this enables the player to repeat the CD or tape over and over again).

Regardless of what form of anesthesia you're receiving during the operation, you can usually wear headphones. However, if the surgery involves your head area in any way, you'd need permission from your surgical team to have the music played overhead during the operation.

ഇളാളെ

JANET'S STORY:
PUTTING MIND-BODY TECHNIQUES TO WORK

Janet, a vivacious forty-seven-year-old woman with a thriving business as a hairstylist, came to see me one day after she'd had an abnormal Pap test. This test is used for the early detection of cancer and other abnormalities of the female genital tract, especially of the cervix. This was the third time a Pap test had indicated the presence of precancerous cells, and the cells on her latest biopsy looked even more irregular than they had on previous occasions.

Janet had two teenage children and was not planning future pregnancies. For these reasons, I recommended a vaginal hysterectomy. I also felt that she would benefit from an intensive nutritional and lifestyle program. Beyond removing the renegade cells, I wanted to assist her in addressing their root cause. Together we explored how she might quit smoking and how, in addition to a whole-foods-based diet, she might benefit from our Power Healing Drink (see recipe, page 73) and supplementation with antioxidants. She started this regimen the month before surgery.

Two weeks before the operation, we developed a self-hypnosis script for her to use with imagery of a tropical lagoon and a cleansing waterfall. She visualized herself standing under the waterfall and all toxins and aberrant cells being washed away. She recorded the tape herself and listened to it lying in bed for 15 minutes each night before falling asleep.

After the surgery, Janet felt surprisingly calm and relatively free of pain. At the hospital, a friend who was a massage therapist came to give her a gentle total body lymphatic massage to let her own "internal cleansing waterfall" support her healing. At home, she prepared an herbal rinse to let go on a spiritual level. A wonderful herbalist in my town, Suki Roth, grows and blends a selection of herbs for these herbal baths. The combination, which includes comfrey, holy basil, and other herbs, is brewed into a bath rinse to help clear the emotional and spiritual trauma. This was particularly helpful in Janet's case because she was a survivor of childhood sexual abuse. I wanted to make sure that her surgery became an empowering experience of renewal rather than an assault on her well-being. Janet told me that the herbal bath was profoundly soothing, and she had felt her fears and anxieties dissolving away with each successive rinse.

Janet was back to work as a hairstylist in record time. Her Pap smears over the last three years have been completely normal. She has given up smoking and continues to eat a low-fat, vegetable-rich diet, along with taking a balanced multiple designed to support women's health. Emotionally, she has reclaimed a sense of peace and wholeness in her daily life. I feel confident that Janet's salubrious lifestyle will help her to stave off cancer and will continue to do so in the future.

—EGM

❧ The Broader Context of Surgical Success

As we've discussed, what happens in the operating room may be just as critical to your healing process after surgery as what happens before and after the operation. Beyond music and healing suggestions there are other factors that can influence your body's ability to mend after the experience of surgery. These include the surgical technique, temperature, oxygen availability, and massage.

Surgical technique. While a certain degree of injury is inevitable, the type of surgery *and* the surgical techniques used will also have a major impact on your recovery time. Open-heart surgery, for example, requires a much longer recovery time than, say, finger surgery or a vasectomy. Surgical techniques, too, are a key factor in how quickly you will mend. Your surgeon will attempt to minimize trauma to the tissues by creating incisions with a scalpel and reserving scissors for dissection. He or she will try to make the operation proceed as smoothly and efficiently as possible, thereby minimizing exposure to the tissues below your skin. Longer exposure heightens the risks of infection and desiccation (drying out of tissue), and these, too, can delay the healing process. There are many other aspects of surgical technique that can lessen your body's stress burden and improve your recovery after surgery. A skilled surgeon will exploit these techniques to the greatest extent possible. Also, many procedures can now be performed using minimally invasive techniques such as laparoscopy, hysteroscopy, or arthroscopy. These less invasive techniques involve smaller incisions and shorter recovery times. Check with your surgeon to see if they have training in minimally invasive techniques or if they can refer you to someone with skill in this type of procedure.

Temperature. Environmental conditions, too, can affect your rate of healing after surgery. It is known, for example, that wounds heal more quickly at warmer temperatures than at a normal room temperature of 18 to 20°C. Cold temperatures can actually impair the wound healing process. Patients undergoing major surgery frequently experience a drop in body temperature (hypothermia). Research has also shown that the rate of gain of tensile strength—or how strong the new tissue is—in wounds decreases by about 20 percent when the wound area is exposed to 12°C.[37] Weight loss and protein losses may be higher at cooler ambient temperatures and cold or coolness in general causes a constriction of blood vessels limiting the blood supply to the wound.[38]

One solution is *active warming,* using such strategies as warmed intravenous fluids and warming of the skin.[39] Active warming before and during surgery reduces the risk of infections, supports normal healing, and shortens hospitalization time.[40] You may want to see if the anesthetist will be able to provide an air warming blanket. This can help reduce your risk of prolonged bleeding and infection, and of needing additional anesthesia.

Also, after the initial period of intense inflammation (during which a cold press or ice may be helpful) has subsided, a heat lamp in the vicinity of your surgical wound might actually accelerate the healing process.[41] Consult with your physician before using this strategy for your particular situation. At a minimum, a warm and comfortable environment during surgery is important, and the occasional, moderate use of external heat may further accelerate healing.

Oxygen. During and after surgery, all tissues require an adequate supply of oxygen to heal well and to prevent complications of infection.[42] Oxygen is an important cell signal that interacts with growth factors to accelerate wound healing.[43] It's needed for cell metabolism and for the formation of new *collagen,* the basic protein that binds or holds together new tissue. Also, immune cells need oxygen to help with the wound-healing process. The processes of proliferation and migration of cells, which eventually enable "sealing" of the wound (epithelialization), are also oxygen-dependent.

Blood, of course, is the main vehicle for oxygen and other nutrients. This is why you need to make sure that you have good blood circulation around the wound area. As a wise old surgeon friend once told us, "Wounds that do not bleed are wounds that typically will not heal." Specific nutrients such as the amino acid L-arginine, a widely available supplement, can be helpful in promoting oxygen transfer to tissues. L-arginine apparently works by increasing nitric oxide production, which in turn dilates the blood vessels and enhances blood flow.

Another oxygen-boosting supplement is organic germanium. Drs. Keith Berend and Adolph Lombardi of Joint Implant Surgeons in Columbus, Ohio, include germanium as an integral part of their "holistic peri-operative, rapid-recovery program" for patients having either total hip or total knee replacement (arthroplasty).[44] This program, which includes various dietary supplements and post-op rehabilitation, has led to a significantly decreased length of hospital stay and significantly lower hospital readmission rates for patients who have these orthopedic surgeries.[45] The mechanism by which germanium increases the body's oxygen supply is not entirely clearly. One theory is that germanium may facilitate the entry of oxygen into red blood cells and then enhances the release of oxygen into tissues for faster healing.[46] When purchasing germanium from a reputable source, make sure that it's organic and not inorganic germanium, because only the organic form is safe to take as a supplement.

Oxygen is routinely provided following major surgery, especially when your blood circulation is poor. It's usually administered through the nose, using a *nasal canula* or via a face mask.[47] This strategy is increasingly used for those who are kept overnight and for those suffering from sleep apnea (difficulty breathing) or respiratory weaknesses. Massage, too, can be helpful to improve circulation and oxygen delivery to help with healing (see below).

—High-Tech Oxygen Delivery—

Hyperbaric oxygen therapy, or HBOT, seems to enhance wound healing in situations where the blood supply to the wound area is very poor and thus oxygen is lacking.[48] Hyperbaric oxygen refers to oxygen delivered in a specially constructed chamber at an atmospheric pressure higher than the pressure at sea level. One study shows that for people with foot ulcers due to diabetes, HBOT significantly increases the healing potential of the wounds.[49] By reducing the complications of infection, this therapy also helps diabetic patients avoid the need for foot amputation.[50] The approach seems particularly effective when an anaerobic infection is present.[51] Despite its relatively high cost, HBOT seems justified when available, at least for people with diabetic foot infections.

Manipulation and massage. Gentle touch or therapeutic massage can be helpful in getting your blood circulation going after surgery, and this, in turn, can help prevent the formation of dangerous blood clots. For certain procedures, your surgeon may administer stocking and compression booties during surgery to prevent blood clots from occurring in your legs. These will be placed in the operating room and worn until you can walk fully after surgery. They will give your legs a nice massage. Do not be surprised if you awaken after surgery with these types of boots on—especially if you are having orthopedic or major abdominal or pelvic surgery. In general, take steps to ensure good blood circulation in the area of the wound and in your legs when you're bedridden. Massage, movement (bicycle motion if you're in bed), low-fat diet, and avoiding tight bandages—all can help improve circulation. Osteopathic manipulation is also very helpful in restoring function after surgery.

ᔈᕀ Whole-Body Relaxation Sequences for Rapid Repair and Recovery

A key part of any healing plan is the reduction of both real and perceived stress. To keep stress in check, consider taping the following scripts, which can be read by you or a loved one. Listen to any of the scripts or parts of the scripts that appeal to you before, during, and after surgery. Listen to your tape with headphones to remove outside noise or play some quiet calming music in the background when you're making your tape

What follows are three of the scripts we use for our patients around the time of surgery. The mind-body relaxation script includes progressive muscle relaxation as well as some guided imagery and several self-hypnotic suggestions for healing. You can use it to decrease stress, increase the relaxation response, and promote a faster, more comfortable and uncomplicated recovery. It's not necessary to become totally unconscious during the relaxation tape, but a "relaxed readiness" will help you gain some degree of control over what happens to you, and this alone can help you feel calmer. The pain relief script uses guided imagery and mindful breathing to diminish pain. The script for healing combines hypnotic suggestions with guided imagery and relaxation to promote relaxation before surgery, optimal body-mind conditions during surgery, and rapid recovery after surgery.

Before listening to the scripts, make sure your clothes are fitting comfortably and go to a place where you won't be disturbed for 20 to 30 minutes.

BODY-MIND RELAXATION SCRIPT

Get yourself into a comfortable position, sitting or lying where you can safely go into a relaxed state. You are now going to be able to put yourself into a deeply relaxing, health-promoting and healing space.

Start by taking three slow, deep conscious breaths, in and out. Gently close your eyes if that feels comfortable to you. Imagine a healing place for yourself. In your mind see yourself in a beautiful place—some place where you can feel at peace and completely accepted, perhaps a place in nature—a hammock under a palm tree by a soothing sea, for example. See, hear, and feel yourself resting and recovering in this healing place.

This is your special place. You can go there any time by closing your eyes and taking a breath. If you have trouble visualizing then just feel yourself held in a warm healing light. From your special place, we will start counting slowly backward from 20. Count down with each breath, allowing tension in your muscles and worry to wash away with each exhalation.

20—Now just let your body begin to unwind.

19—Relaxing body and mind.

18—Relaxing body, mind, and spirit.

17—Maybe you are already noticing how much more relaxed you can feel.

16—Perhaps already feeling places in your body softening more and more. Allow your scalp muscles to relax. You may experience a slight tingling sensation in your scalp. Or you might feel the deep relaxing of your scalp muscles as they begin to spread and flow. Relaxation flowing down across your eyes, down across your face. Relax your cheek and jaw muscles. Roll your eyes gently up to your eyebrows. Stretch your jaw open and closed.

15—A quarter of the way down and you're already feeling your neck and shoulder muscles lengthening more and more. Let your breath go gently into any tight spot. Begin to really enjoy your relaxation and comfort.

14—Now relax the chest, abdomen, and thighs, let the breath deepen and fill these areas, just let go and feel peaceful and comfortable.

13—Relax more and more with the sound of each number, and even allow any distracting sounds to become a part of your experience of comfort and relaxation.

12—As you allow the relaxation to spread, notice the peaceful, restful, and comfortable warmth or coolness spreading down into your shoulders, into your arms. You may notice one arm feeling heaver than the other. Perhaps your arms feel pleasantly light or comfortably heavy. Perhaps both feel equally comfortable.

11—Breathe slowly and deeply. Notice the calm beginning to spread as you continue to experience the pleasant, restful relaxation spreading through your body, down through your back, pelvis, hips, legs, and out the soles of your feet.

10—Halfway to the bottom, you can now double your relaxation by breathing deeper. Feel more and more comfortable as you relax deeper and deeper, letting go of all tension.

9—Feeling pleasantly restful, continue to notice the growing, spreading, comfort through your body, mind, and spirit.

8—At times you may hear the tape loud and clear, and at other times it may seem to be a long distance away.

7—Maybe your mind is wandering from time to time and from place to place on other things, as you are filling with a healing tranquillity more and more.

6—Enjoy this relaxation and comfort as you go deeper and deeper.

5—Three quarters of the way down, you're deeper and deeper relaxed as your body seems to just sink down deeper and deeper.

4—Wondering perhaps what to expect at the count of one, but realizing it will be a pleasant healing experience.

3—Already becoming more and more relaxed. Continue to enjoy your experience of comfortable relaxation.

2—Almost to the bottom as you continue to go deeper and deeper as you breathe, slowly, comfortably, and peacefully.

1—Nothing to disturb you, feeling more and more comfortable, deeply, deeply relaxed. Deeper with each breath that you take, with each sound you hear. Deeply, deeply relaxed.

Now that the mind, body, and spirit are in a fully tranquil state, we will start to plant the seed of healing. A seed that is planted in the soil instinctively knows how to grow. It knows how to obtain nutrients and water from the soil, and energy from the sun. It knows how to breathe. It trusts the careful gardener to care for it. When a flower or fruit is picked the plant knows how to heal over. It will constrict the flow of sap and form a new layer or cells. Unconsciously it will thrive into a robust healthy plant.

All living creatures unconsciously know how to heal. With your unconscious mind your body can easily and quickly heal from illness or surgery. With your unconscious body-mind you can return to full strength, superb function, and well-being. Like the plant, your body knows how to stop unnecessary bleeding and quickly heal any tissue injury with the good nutrients you can supply your body. Using your ability to do slow, deep breathing, you can help your body release endorphins and other healing substances to prevent discomfort, nausea, or infection. By closing your eyes and picturing your special place, you can be free of anxiety. Like careful gardeners, your caregivers will carefully and skillfully nurture your ability to heal. Your body is ready to heal to a radiant full health. Breathe in the relaxation that comes from knowing that you are healing every day.

Now that you have been to your healing place it is time to come back to your daily life. As you count back up from 1 to 20, you will return slowly and fully to a state of usual awareness, but be able to maintain a sense of peace and relaxation. Gently count back up from one to twenty.. Gradually open your eyes and feel refreshed and ready.

PAIN RELIEF SCRIPT

Take a relaxing position. Prepare to gently close your eyes. Your eyelids can start to feel heavy. You may want to let them drop. As they get heavier, you can anticipate a heavy wave of warmth that may float down through your body when they close. As they get heavier, gently close them and feel the wave of warm relaxation spread over you. Now allow that relaxation to spread to the breath.

Take a slow deep relaxing breath in to the count of 3, pause for the count of 3, and then let the breath out to the count of 5.

Breath in 2 3
Pause 2 3
Out 2 3 4 5
Breath in 2 3
Pause 2 3
Out 2 3 4 5

Feel yourself relaxing and going deeper with each breath. Now with this slow steady breath in the background imagine you hear the slow relaxing sound of the ocean on the beach . . . rolling in and out . . . a lovely beach with a gentle breeze. Maybe you are rocking in a comfortable hammock under some palm trees listening to the sound of the ocean waves. The light is soft and clear, the temperature is perfectly comfortable. The air is clean and fresh . . . rocking back and forth. You may be at peace. You look out at the sea. It is your sea of comfort, pain relief, and anesthesia. Your sea is a beautiful soothing and relieving color. You can start by walking over to the sea. Just for the moment, imagine dipping you hand into that ocean and taking a really big handful of it. . . . Can you feel that in your hand? Is it warm or cool? . . . Good. . . . Now, in your mind, just rub the liquid gently into any area of discomfort. . . . Can you feel a wave of tingling comfort? Now feel the pain steadily diminishing. . . . Okay, that's good. . . . Rinsing away the pain that used to be in your body . . . doesn't that feel good! . . . Right, now let's do all that again. . . . Dip in and fill another handful of that healing numbing fluid and gently rub it in. . . . Now, what's happening this time? This time the comfort and pleasure can double. Repeat the application as many times as you like until all the pain is gone or any pain that left is so diminished that it's of no great consequence. Enter the sea of comfort and swim and float in a blissful buoyant anesthesia for as long as you like. The pleasure and comfort is spreading through you body. The more you feel the ocean holding and supporting you the more comfort you will be able to feel.

Good, you did that beautifully. Now, you can do that whenever you need to. . . . Just relax yourself as much as you can then do exactly the same thing that we've done today. . . . And do you know, each time you do that, the benefit will last even longer!

All right, now it's time to bring the tape to an end, just knowing that ocean of healing is always there for you, whenever you need it. . . . Let's repeat the breathing sequence from the beginning to bring you back. You will return fresh and ready.

Breath in 2 3 you are returning to consciousness
Pause 2 3
Out 2 3 4 5

You are back fresh and comfortable to meet the day ahead.

SCRIPT FOR HEALING

This script is divided into three sections: creating a healing space, envisioning a successful surgery, and visualizing a speedy recovery. The first two sections are most helpful before and during the surgery (if you're going to be awake). If you have time, you can get a head start on the recovery phase by listening to all three sections. In the post-op period, you may want to listen mostly to the last section.

Part 1: Your Healing Space

Take a comfortable position sitting or lying down. Relax and allow that relaxation to spread to the breath. Take a few nice long slow deep breaths in and slowly breathe out. . . . Notice that with each breath you feel more and more calm. . . . Now once again take a long slow, slow deep breath in and out. Notice how you are beginning to relax. Take another slow deep breath . . . in and out. Notice how much more relaxed you are. . . . Prepare to gently close your eyes. Your eyelids can start to feel heavy. As they get heavier, you can anticipate a heavy wave of warmth that may float down through your body when they close. Again, take a long slow, slow deep breath and this time, when you exhale, your eyes close naturally as you . . . relax deeply.

As your eyes gently close, feel the wave of warm relaxation spread over you. Notice how much more relaxed you are now. Continue to breathe normally and naturally. Let each and every breath you take relax you more and more. . . . Allow yourself to drift into a peaceful state. . . . Relaxing can be pleasurable.

We will start by creating your own safe healing space. Imagine you are on a holiday and you are walking to your safe healing space. You are free of all responsibilities and cares. You are walking through a beautiful forest of redwoods and ferns. The light is soft, and temperature comfortable. You enter a beautiful glade and see a beautiful clear stream running near a mossy wildflower garden. You can smell the delicate scent of the flowers. Carry on walking along the path . . . until you reach a decorative white footbridge . . . which passes over the stream. You can hear the water as it splashes over the stones . . . making a rippling sound. You cross the bridge and enter a healing place. You are surrounded by healing light. Bask in this healing relaxing light for as along as you want. Between the trees is a soft inviting hammock. Lie down and rock gently in the hammock, bathed in the healing light. Do this whenever you need to escape to a healing, loving, and safe place.

You are now able to easily relax on your command. With your own breath, you can relax. With your own imagination you can travel to your safe relaxing place. With your own body and mind you can restore yourself to wellness. Every time you hear the phrase, "You are moving toward health," all of your systems come together to function in a normal healthy manner. . . . They create complete recovery within and without. . . . Relax, take a deep breath. . . . You are moving toward health. . . . Let yourself sink deeper and deeper into a peaceful relaxed state.

Part 2

In your imagination, begin rehearsing for your successful surgical procedure in a safe and relaxed way. It is safe and enjoyable to be this relaxed. Through the power of your mind's eye you can see yourself walking into the surgical center. You walk with confidence, you speak with relaxed self-assurance, and you smile. . . . You say to yourself, "This is where I am going to get healthy. . . . This is where my body is going to be repaired so it can get well. . . . This is where I can go to help my doctor help me to ease my body. . . . I make the decisions for my well being. . . . I have decided that this is a surgery that will bring my body to wellness and wholeness. . . . The surgeon and staff are here to support me. . . . We are a team."

[Take a few moments to rest into your imagination.]

Good, you're now moving toward health. You have equanimity and peace about your decisions. Thoughts and feelings can come and go. You are in control of what you think and feel. You can just let go of any thoughts or fears. Good, you are doing fine. . . . Each and every time you practice this, you become calmer and more relaxed. What we picture in the imagination can become reality. You are creating, through a positive attitude the image of complete recovery.

Now let the scene change to the room where the procedure is to take place. You are feeling relaxed and poised. Let it happen. You're doing fine. Your doctor is there to help bring your body, mind, and spirit into full integration and peace. You relax even deeper as the anesthetic is administered. Because of your deep relaxation, you only need a very small amount of anesthetic to get your body ready for the procedure and to keep you at the perfect level of comfort.

You are moving toward health. You can hear noises around you, but you pay no attention to them. . . . The scene changes . . . back to the safe place. You find yourself in the hammock. Rocking in it has a nice steady rhythm and you feel calm and relaxed as you look out onto your stream and woods of peace. . . . Calm and tranquil . . . enjoying the scene that is before you. Feeling the rhythm of the hammock, smelling the aromas and scents of nature, enjoying the sun on the water . . . calm and tranquil . . . calm and tranquil . . . calm and tranquil . . . Your body cooperates with the skillful hands of the surgeon. It opens up easily, it has only the exact amount of blood flow that is necessary to maintain health. . . . In fact your body knows exactly what to do, and it does it in perfect concert with the surgeon. . . . All of your vital signs are in perfect order: blood pressure perfect, heart rate steady, breathing normal. You are enjoying your time in the safe place, calm . . . and relaxed . . . calm and tranquil. You are moving toward health. . . .

Interestingly enough, from the very moment that you decided to have this surgery; your body began the healing process. . . . Your body knows just what to do in order to get you to wellness. All of your blood cells are doing their job carrying oxygen, preventing infection, clearing inflammation. . . . The healing system is on automatic, the immune system is functioning perfectly, and everything about you is working with your medical team. . . . They are doing the job that is theirs to do, while your healing system and immune system are doing their work. . . . Take a few moments to let these suggestions take complete effect upon you. . . .

[One minute pause.]

You are doing fine. . . .

You are aware that a procedure has taken place. You can feel a little pressure, but that is all. Any discomfort is minimal and you are full of energy. . . . You are in control and healing has begun and will continue.

If you are listening to this in preparation for the procedure, you may open your eyes now, knowing that you have created a new healthy future waiting for your body and mind to manifest. If you are using this during the surgical procedure continue to stay at your healing place until you hear that it is time to awaken . . . when the anesthetist is saying your name, and not before, come to full wakeful consciousness. Notice how relaxed and comfortable you feel.

Part 3

Begin to envision how quickly you will recover. You are moving toward health. When you awaken from your procedure, you have an appetite and can eat small amounts of food, easily and effortlessly. You find that you are thirsty and can drink water easily. Your bladder and bowel can work easily and effortlessly. All of your organs are functioning normally and naturally. Over the next weeks your whole metabolism becomes tuned into your individual needs. You digest your food easily and limit the quantities so that you're eating just the right amount of nutritious food. You desire only the foods that are good for you. And because you are becoming so much calmer inside, you feel a sense of acceptance, a feeling of peace and serenity deep within you.

Your metabolism during your resting periods becomes much more natural and is adjusted for your relaxed state and, because of all these improvements to your system, your heartbeat becomes steadier and your breathing becomes effortless. Because of the increased oxygen intake in your lungs, your autonomic nervous system, which controls your heart rate and your breathing, is working in peace and harmony. Because of the improved nervous system, your digestion and kidneys begin to function more effectively and you feel a tremendous improvement to your entire being. The blood supply to your vital organs such as your liver, your pancreas, and your spleen will nourish these organs more effectively as all the chemistry in your body becomes more balanced and stable.

Your brain waves are becoming steady, and this indicates a more peaceful and restful state of being. Because of this, you're sleeping more soundly and having beautiful dreams. When you wake up, you feel refreshed, invigorated, and fully alert.

Your improved biochemical and metabolic system causes your general resistance to infections and diseases to improve. You begin to return to your normal activities with focus and energy.

The muscle tone improves and you have more vigor with which to carry out your daily tasks, your complexion and hair radiate vitality from within. And all these things are beginning to take place deep within you, right now. You have completed your journey toward health.

When the time is right, just open your eyes feeling ready, knowing that you are repairing and recovering. You create your own reality. Today, your reality is that of a relaxed healthy human being, feeling balanced in body, mind, and spirit.

These scripts comprise some of the tools you may want to use to shore up your healing process. Feel free to vary them to fit your individual needs.

❧ Getting the Support You Need, Beginning with Your Surgical Team

There are many ways you can feel supported as you prepare for surgery. On a very pragmatic level, the first place to look for support is in your relationship with your surgical team. You need to feel confident about the skills and knowledge of the various members of your team—the physicians, nurses, and technicians to whom you've entrusted your life. Ideally, everyone on your surgical team should be willing to listen to your concerns and to then patiently and respectfully answer your questions. You deserve as much, because after all, *they work for you.* They should be responsive to your needs in ways that leave you feeling comfortable and secure. If this is not the case, then talk to your surgeon and see if you can arrive at some happy middle ground between your expectations and reality. If you decide that your surgeon's attitude and bedside manner just don't sit well with you, then try communicating with others on the surgical team who may be more attentive to your needs.

A pre-op visit to the hospital will give you additional time to meet with other members of the team, including the nurses, anesthesiologist, and nurse anesthetist. Make sure there's at least one person on the team who you feel communicates well and supports you on a personal psychological level. Let that person know how much you appreciate him or her. If you generally feel positive about your surgical team, be sure to voice your confidence in them. This kind of communication is likely to enhance the tenor of the experience for all involved.

Beyond trying to cultivate a positive relationship with your surgical team, having a good support team outside of the hospital or clinic is equally important. Friends and family are usually are our first allies, but think carefully about who can support you through the experience. Try to give yourself sufficient time to extend invitations and assemble your team. When you offer the invitation, make sure that you make your expectations clear, in a gentle and appreciative way, from the beginning. You may be surprised to learn that friends and relatives feel honored and delighted to help you in any way they can; nonetheless, they will also need to be clear and okay with your personal expectations.

To assist you with this communication, here are some of the roles that might be assigned to different members of your support team.

Home-based support. This team member would attend to a variety of domestic duties, helping to organize and execute daily life tasks that need to be taken care of while you are away from home or convalescing—responsibilities such as the mail, bills, child care, pet care, plant care, recycling, and cleaning the house. Having someone come in to care for your children or pets while you recover enables you to focus more energy on your own healing, which should be your first priority following the surgery.

Dietary support. Several team members can help arrange for food to be brought to you in the hospital and after you return home. Try to get someone or perhaps several friends to help you prepare meals in advance, so that when you return home, you don't need to cook. Some grocery stores and restaurants make home deliveries. Getting meals together will not come easily if you're feeling nauseous and weak during this time, so having this kind of support can be invaluable. Preparing food and freezing it ahead of time, and having your favorite comfort foods available in the days and weeks after the surgery can be a wonderful gift.

Logistical support. This team member would help you arrange your home for your return by moving furniture or arranging to rent special equipment you might need. Make sure that your bed has easy access to a phone. Also, think about your needs in terms of entertainment, from books and videos to artistic activities and games you can play while you're recuperating. You may want to have your team member rent you some upbeat, funny, or soothing videos, or to borrow them from friends.

Advocacy support. As part of this team approach, consider asking a friend or relative to act as an *advocate*. This individual would be able to make health care decisions on your behalf. To formalize this relationship, you may want to sign an advanced health care directive or durable power of attorney for health care. This type of legal document is especially necessary if you do not have a recognized legal relationship with your partner. Decide if you want a partner, parents, or other relatives to be legally in charge. Make sure to clarify your wishes with your advocate regarding advanced life support, organ donation, and what you would want done under differing surgical scenarios. Set up a will, a living will, if you haven't done so already. Again, your advocate will have backup documents clarifying your wishes in any of the surgical scenarios mentioned above. If you're not in a legal marriage and your partner is serving as the advocate, make sure that your wishes are legally documented.

We urge you to bring along your advocate when you meet with your doctors before the surgery. He or she essentially serves as a contact person who will relay information about the outcome of the surgery and how you are doing until you are ready to take over that responsibility. This person should be someone who can help you communicate clearly with your health care team, including taking notes during the doctors' meetings so that you don't have to worry about remembering everything. If at all possible, have your advocate stay with you for the entire time you are in the hospital. Hospital errors are all too common, and many can be prevented or minimized with vigilance; caring friends and relatives will often notice subtle changes that busy nurses or physicians miss. To this end, your advocate is someone who should be assertive and persistent on your behalf if needed.

Ideally, the person you choose for this role should be someone who feels stable, aware, attentive, and calming to you—someone with whom you feel comfortable discussing your deepest concerns as well as your pettiest ones. He or she may be able to help you address specific fears well in advance of the surgery by helping you obtain information, by accompanying you on a hospital tour, or by helping you contact another person who has had this surgery already who could talk to you and allay your fears. Your advocate may also be called upon to help you practice some of the techniques presented in this chapter.

Beyond your personal support team, you might also consider working with a counselor or psychotherapist. This individual can help you work through any anger, irritation, or frustration related to your situation, or toward the body part that "isn't working right." This, too, must be someone you feel you can trust, someone who gives you permission to express your feelings, and someone who can gently guide you toward deep emotional releases. Remember that the more you can bring your inner conflicts to the surface and work through them, the more peaceful you will feel. In addition, some forms of bodywork can, in the context of psychotherapy, help release repressed emotions at a level beyond words and normal cognitive functioning.[52]

A good counselor also can help you resolve guilt around past behaviors that may have resulted in the need for surgery. Learning to appreciate and accept your body with compassion for all of its flaws and forgiving yourself for any mistakes that you have made will bring you a sense of self acceptance, a key step toward healing. If you don't feel that a therapist is in order, then simply give voice to your fears and worries with your surgeon or with an empathetic friend.

After the surgery, you may want to join or form a support group, at least during the initial phases of your recovery. This could be an informal support group consisting of two or three friends who are surgical veterans. It might simply be a meditation group, in which people cultivate inner calm by sitting together in silence, or you may elect to join a more formal support group, one that deals specifically with your particular condition (for example, a breast cancer support group). If you do this, make sure the group truly supports you in ways that feel comfortable to you. Not all support groups are run well, and some may provide a better fit for you than others.

One other aspect of support that you may want to consider is prayer. Depending on your religious outlook, prayer may be an appropriate adjunct to your recovery. You may experience a profound sense of well being as you receive the loving thoughts and meditations of members of a prayer group. Although the data are somewhat conflicting, self-prayer and prayer by another person (intercessory prayer) in several studies have been shown aid in healing.[53] We still don't really know how prayer works. A recent randomized trial suggests that prayer is more likely to promote healing in those who sincerely believe in its power.[54]

The take-home lesson for those who prefer prayer is this: There's no harm in asking people who care about you to send you prayers or positive thoughts during the time of your operation and afterward. There may even be a substantial benefit. Another option is to arrange for a spiritual adviser or a religious leader from your church to pray for you or to visit you in the hospital. At the very least, we know that praying quietly yourself before and after surgery can help allay fears and put you in a calmer frame of mind.

This brings us to the spiritual side of surgery. Major surgery is often a time when people experience a "wake-up call" to reevaluate their life's direction and priorities. Prior to surgery, you may want to consult a spiritual adviser or counselor about this emergent awareness or any existential fears or questions you may have.[55] You may also want to do some journaling (simply writing down your thoughts and feelings, as if you are writing a letter to yourself) to determine what meaning this surgery has for you. Some patients have told us that they found it very helpful to have their pastor or hospital chaplain pay a visit while they're recuperating.

❧ A Gentle Reminder

Try to keep in mind—clearly and calmly—that the fight-or-flight stress response not only causes your heart to race and blood pressure to rise, it also suppresses immunity and suspends tissue repair and healing. You have it within your power not to succumb to the more oppressive, destructive side of stress. By limiting tension and anxiety and increasing your body's ability to mount the relaxation response, you will facilitate your own healing. You will be setting yourself up for a more harmonious and expedient recovery.

Although surgery can be stressful, there are many ways to help you cope. The various relaxation techniques we have shared in this chapter can clearly benefit your body's healing response to surgery. Any one or combination of the self-regulation strategies can help bolster your mind's resilience and adaptability.

They can be used to either direct health-promoting, life-enhancing messages to the body or to simply induce states of inner tranquillity and well-being.

Relaxed readiness, concentration on a positive outcome, faith in your health care team, and clear communication—all of these factors can aid in your recovery. Your inner life plays a vital role in healing. Yes, surgical techniques are important, but the body ultimately heals itself. By exploring the various strategies we've laid out in this chapter and creating a solid support network, you will help bring body, mind, and spirit into a harmonious collaboration, and you will better realize your full healing potential.

6

Preventing Postoperative Complications

How poor are they that have not
patience! What wound would ever heal
but by degree?

—Shakespeare, *Othello*

Laurel M., age thirty-five, first learned that she had uterine fibroids in
2002. Laurel sought medical advice from me to find out about therapies that
might help reduce her monthly discomfort and heavy periods. She and her
husband had been trying to conceive for the preceding two years, so the link
between fibroids and infertility was a major concern. She initially hoped to
avoid surgery if at all possible.

We worked together to devise a treatment plan involving specific dietary
changes and supplements, including an antioxidant multiple, omega-3 fatty
acids, and a Chinese herb called tripterygium. She decreased her intake of
dairy and saturated fats and increased fiber and cabbage-family vegetables,
such as broccoli, cauliflower, and Brussels sprouts. She also tried mind-body
approaches, such as mindful breathing, to decrease stress. She began receiving a gentle form of bodywork called craniosacral therapy. At first these

methods seemed helpful and the fibroid symptoms abated for a while. Six months later, however, the fibroids began growing again. Her uterus continued to expand to the point where she looked five months pregnant. Her long, heavy periods interfered with her work as a karate instructor, and she continued to have difficulty becoming pregnant.

One day Laurel told me that she had reached her limit. The pain had become too intense for several days each month, and her biological clock was ticking down the time she had left to have a child. She was ready to have the fibroids removed, a surgery known as myomectomy. This procedure is commonly used when the woman doesn't want a hysterectomy or wishes to preserve her fertility. Like a hysterectomy, however, the myomectomy does entail cutting into the abdomen under general anesthesia. Women typically end up spending about three days in the hospital, and then require several months for a full recovery. Blood loss from the operation can be substantial. (Fortunately, myomectomy is now increasingly performed with a less-extensive procedure called laparoscopic surgery.)

Laurel knew her body was capable of healing from surgery, but she wanted to know if there were any strategies that might help her heal faster, and with the least amount of pain and loss of normal function. Laurel had been maintaining a balanced diet, but I encouraged her to increase her protein and vegetable intake. I then placed her on the Rapid Recovery Supplement regimen and added the Power Healing Drink (see page 73) to her usual routine. Every night for three weeks leading up to the surgery, she listened to a 30-minute relaxation tape her husband had recorded for her.

She also burned a CD of her favorite songs—a mix of Bonnie Raitt, Patsy Cline, and some New Age Celtic music. We played this music during her surgery and carefully counseled everyone to use positive language in the OR setting. While she was under anesthesia, she was kept warm and cozy under a warm air blanket.

Several large fibroids were removed during the operation. Laurel went home on the second day and continued her nutritional program. She called me the next day to say she was experiencing a lot of pain and feeling depressed. When I saw her in the office she admitted she had been afraid to use the narcotic pain pills and had been doing a lot around the house out of *frustration toward her lack of mobility. There was no infection or problem with her incision or exam. I talked to her about the importance of post-op pain management and moderation of activity and rest. She agreed to use the narcotic pain meds along with an herbal anti-inflammatory multiple. We also scheduled her for massage and acupuncture treatments. Her pain management was much better over the next few days. When she returned to our clinic a few weeks later, it was clear that she had recovered quickly and comfortably. Her energy and mobility had been restored to normal. In fact, it was difficult convincing her to wait a few more weeks before she returned to her karate teaching.*

We were all very pleased with this outcome, which was certainly remarkable for her particular situation. Normally, it takes about two months to get to the point that Laurel got to in three weeks. Her recovery had seemed to accelerate the moment she began walking around after the operation.

—EGM

The challenges of recovering from surgery begin as soon as you emerge from the operating room. At this point, you may feel weak, groggy, and vulnerable. Your body may still be numb from the anesthesia, and once this wears off, you'll be trying to find ways to manage the pain and inflammation. By taking proper steps to manage these manifestations of surgical stress, you can help your body move more quickly into a healing mode, and you will speed up your recovery in the process.

What do we mean by *surgical stress?* This refers to the hormonal and nervous system changes that occur in your body in response to surgery.[1] Whenever a serious wound is inflicted, as it is in the case of major surgery, your sympathetic nervous system becomes activated, and a number of stress-related hormones are released, such as adrenaline and cortisol. These changes result in the well-known fight-or-flight response: pupils dilate, blood vessels constrict, muscles tense up, heart rate increases, and salt and water are retained. But of course it's the *experience* of all this stress and tension that resonates most with people who have just undergone a major surgery, and that experience can be anything but pleasant.

Let's take a closer look at what's going on in the body during surgical stress. Within minutes of going "under the knife," your pituitary gland pumps out *adrenocorticotrophic hormone,* or ACTH. This hormone, in turn, stimulates the adrenal glands to secrete a group of stress hormones called *glucocorticoids,* the most notorious of which—at least for medical professionals—is *cortisol.* Blood and saliva levels of cortisol tend to peak about 4 to 6 hours from the start of the surgery. Cortisol stimulates the release and breakdown of stored-up fat, carbohydrate, and protein, so that the body can use these fuels for energy.

This ability to quickly use up stored body fuels is likely to be an evolutionary response to serious injury. As a survival mechanism, it would have served two purposes for early humans. First, if a wild beast attacked you or you were threatened by some natural disaster, those stress hormones would have helped you fight or flee after becoming injured. Second, the "burning" of stored nutrients would have enabled you to sustain yourself until your injuries had healed. Remember that any serious injury could make obtaining food more difficult. By using up those stored body fuels and retaining salt and water, there was a better chance of survival without food until repair and healing had taken place. This explains why seriously injured animals, wild or domestic, can go off to a quiet place and not eat or drink for long periods while they heal.

In the context of modern surgery, though, the increased burning of stored fuels has dubious value. After all, when you're sitting in a hospital bed and being fed on demand, there's no need to be using up your nutrient reserves. Nor is there any need for a heightening of muscular readiness. The tension you experience as your adrenaline levels rise only adds to the stress of simply being in the hospital environment—stress that can be exacerbated by extensive lab tests, the presence of an illness, concerns about postoperative complications, or the loss of physical functioning.

Unfortunately, the breakdown of protein, which occurs in response to adrenaline released with surgery, can lead to a host of adverse changes in your overall health. Muscles can deteriorate, immune function can falter, and hormonal mechanisms can run askew. This *catabolism,* or breakdown of vital tissues, is the hallmark of surgical stress. If the catabolic process is short-lived, then recovery can take place more rapidly. But with a more intense and prolonged breakdown process, there's a much greater risk of experiencing complications such as infections or loss of organ function.[2] Those people most at risk of having such complications include smokers, alcoholics, diabetics, obese individuals, the elderly, and anyone who has undergone frequent surgery in the recent past. The longer you remain in bed and inactive, the more rapidly you will break down muscle and lose protein. Such muscle loss is also partly due to high levels of cortisol in your blood and to the inflammatory chemicals that are initially secreted by tissues in the area around a surgical wound—chemicals that produce redness, heat, and swelling. As time goes on, however, cells that circulate throughout the body as well as cells near the wound begin to generate these inflammatory chemicals. Such chronic, systemic inflammation is itself a symptom of surgical stress. Since the muscles store glutamine, a major fuel for the immune system, the loss of muscle results in increased vulnerability to infections in the wake of the surgery.[3]

Fortunately, your body's response to surgery also entails some hormonal changes that counteract the breakdown process. Your pituitary gland releases increased amounts of *growth hormone* in response to surgery. Growth hormone, as we will see later, is among the key factors your body needs to mount an effective healing response: it stimulates protein synthesis and inhibits the breakdown of protein, enabling you to rapidly form new tissue. The amount of growth hormone produced by your pituitary gland is in direct proportion to the severity or invasiveness of your surgery.[4] This is yet another marvelous manifestation of whole-body wisdom: the larger the injury, the more dramatic the healing response the body elicits.

Another expression of whole-body wisdom is the body's production of natural painkilling chemicals in response to surgery. The pituitary gland produces a surge of a natural painkilling chemical called *beta-endorphin* into the bloodstream following surgery. Beta-endorphin is one of the most powerful means the body has for keeping pain in check: it essentially numbs the body from pain. Hypnotherapy and acupuncture are two ways to naturally increase the body's production of beta-endorphins following surgery.[5] Massage, too, has been found to enhance the secretion of endorphins and thereby relieve pain and anxiety.[6] The use of these noninvasive modalities can substantially reduce the need for pain killers like morphine—something that can translate into much better outcomes for those going through major surgery.

To counteract stress postsurgery, use the various relaxation techniques we introduced in chapter 5. Practicing mindful breathing and listening to relaxation tapes can be immensely beneficial in the postoperative period, particularly if you've already returned to the pressures of daily life. Using strategies such as PMR, self-hypnosis, and mindfulness meditation tempers the fight-or-flight response. Doing them right in your hospital bed and at home helps elicit the relaxation response that has been linked with accelerated healing.

You should also become physically active as soon as possible after your operation. Don't be surprised if you experience some rapid improvements in your health within a few days of resuming exercise. Movement is life; movement expedites healing. When an animal is injured or narrowly escapes injury, it will shake. This muscle shaking evidently helps to rapidly remove the toxic stress chemicals from the system. An early return to movement can likewise start to clear lactic acid and other breakdown products from your system. Passive movement with massage can be helpful as well.

In addition, the supplement options described in Table 6.1 can help temper the stress response. This will help enhance your blood and lymph circulation, bolster immunity and detoxification, and stimulate the production of growth hormone, which is needed for optimal tissue repair. Regardless of how you tend to your physical and emotional well-being, it is also helpful to be aware of the seven potential consequences of surgical stress that will require more specific attention on your part.

Table 6.1. Nutriceutical Strategies for Tempering the Stress Response

ANTISTRESS NUTRICEUTICALS	BENEFITS AND PRACTICAL CONSIDERATIONS
Antistress multiple: B vitamins, vitamin C, minerals, small amounts of ginseng and other adaptogen herbs	These stress-fighting supplements are usually labeled as such and include a high concentration of B-complex vitamins. The B vitamins work together as a team to enhance energy levels, mood, and mental functioning. Vitamin C may help preserve adrenal and immune function. Take as directed on the label.

Pantothenic acid (Vitamin B$_5$)	This B vitamin may help maintain healthy adrenal function, restoring cortisol levels after they have bottomed out; 500 mg per day may be therapeutic.
Rhodiola rosea (golden root, Arctic root)	This herb stimulates the nervous system, reduces physical and mental fatigue, and may be especially helpful in reducing depression. Recommended dose is 50 to 250 mg one to three times daily; or 500 mg in the first 3 days following surgery.
Theanine (an amino acid from green tea)	This key component of green tea promotes resilience and relaxation, without causing the grogginess or sedation that is associated with common medications; also may enhance memory. The suggested dose of theanine to induce relaxation is 100 mg; take this dose four times throughout the day for first 2 weeks after surgery.
Holy basil (Ocimum sanctum)	Known as *tulsi* in Ayurveda, this herb may lower cortisol levels and has significant antistress and anti-inflammatory properties; it may help relieve headache; sometimes combined with other stress-mediating herbs like bacopa. Dosages vary widely; take as directed on the label.
Kava and other herbal sedatives (hops, lemongrass, chamomile, valerian, passionflower)	This is a popular herbal sedative, perhaps best used as part of an antistress herbal formula; take 60–120 mg daily of standardized extracts; do not use for longer than 3 months without medical supervision. All of these herbs have well-documented calming and sedative properties; various combinations have been used with some success to relax the body and to encourage more restful sleep at night.

OTHER NATURAL ANTISTRESS AGENTS*

Eleuthero (commonly referred to as Siberian ginseng)	This herb may help improve adrenal function and reduces physical and mental fatigue. During prolonged stress, it may reduce cortisol levels and increase adrenal capacity; when a person is relaxed, it may raise cortisol and generate alertness. Dosages may range from 15 mg to 500 mg. Adults over age 25 may take 1 to 2 grams per day for weeks at a time; longer periods of daily use are not recommended.

Minor bupleurum	This Chinese herb was recently shown to help relieve various stress-related disorders, including prevention and mitigation of panic attacks when combined with the herb dragon bone. Traditional Chinese doctors say that this combination calms the mind and alleviates anxiety. Take as directed on the label.
Inositol/choline blend, often with niacinamide (vitamin B$_3$ amide)	Inositol is required for proper formation of cell membranes and affects nerve transmission; high doses may help prevent panic attacks in susceptible individuals. Niacinamide and choline reinforce the effects of inositol, enhancing resilience; take high-dose inositol only under professional supervision.
Wood betony (betony, purple betony, wild hop)	This herb works as a muscle relaxant; dosages will vary depending on which part of the plant is used and on whether it is an herbal or homeopathic preparation; consult with a knowledgable pratitioner before using.
DHEA	This supplement may help moderate the effects of high cortisol levels; people with adrenal insufficiency and low DHEA-S may benefit from 50 mg daily of DHEA. Use of 7-KETO DHEA is safer because it avoids the undesirable increases in sex steroids resulting from DHEA supplementation.

---

*Please consult with a qualified health care professional before deciding on dosages and combinations of these supplements. Some supplements taken in incorrect doses or for too long a duration can weaken or suppress the function of your adrenal glands.

❧ Potential Consequences of Surgical Stress— and What to Do About Them

The care that you receive in the first hours and days after surgery plays a crucial role in minimizing the risk of surgical stress-related problems. In this section, we provide you with practical guidance for preventing or alleviating such complications as blood clots, diarrhea, pneumonia, or even heart attacks. In addition to helping you deal with these potential emergencies, we will show you how to deal with more common problems, such as nausea, vomiting, fluid balance, and pain control.

Despite all the technological advances that have been made in medicine over the past few decades, we have yet to solve the problem of surgical stress. The body's responses to being deeply cut can lead to a host of complications or serious physical problems that medical professionals refer to as *morbidity*. It's important to be aware of the possibility for these undesirable aftereffects because they can seriously hamper your ability to heal and make a smooth recovery.

Your body's response to surgical stress is complex and involves far more than just the sympathetic nervous system. The hormonal and metabolic systems are also intimately involved, and many of the outward consequences of surgical stress result from the excessive activation of these systems as well. Indeed, almost all organ systems may be affected.[7]

The seven main complications arising from surgical stress are discussed below.

1. Cardiac overload. When your sympathetic nervous system is activated in response to surgical stress, your heart rate increases and peripheral blood vessels constrict, resulting in increased blood pressure. At the same time, blood vessels around the heart constrict, and this reduces the blood and oxygen supply to the heart muscles, thereby boosting the risk of heart failure or heart attack. If you have a history of coronary artery disease or if you're at risk for heart disease, you may be more susceptible to cardiac complications of this kind.[8]

Stress management techniques and cardiorespiratory fitness training before the surgery can help you reduce the cardiac burden of surgical stress. Also helpful are a low-fat, high-fiber diet and use of supplements that can be taken daily for one month prior to surgery in order to provide additional support for a healthier, more resilient heart: coenzyme Q10 (60 to 120 milligrams per day), fish oil (1 to 3 grams per day), garlic (1 to 2 cloves per day), and hawthorn berry (1 to 2 tablets of the standardized extract per day).[9] Remember that garlic and fish oil should be stopped one week before surgery. Hawthorn is an herbal tonic that has been used successfully since the late 19th century to relieve circulatory insufficiency, symptoms of heart failure, and various other cardiovascular problems.[10]

Fluid balance is very important to maintaining good cardiac function. The anesthesia and nursing staff will carefully monitor any blood or fluid loss due to open wounds or burns and replace it with intravenous fluids or blood transfusions if needed. In the days leading up to surgery, remember to drink plenty of water unless your surgeon recommends otherwise. If you're required to have a bowel cleansing preparation before abdominal surgery, drink extra water to make up for any losses of fluid.

After surgery, your surgeon will want to carefully monitor your fluid balance. Urine output is a good indication of hydration, heart and kidney function, and fluid balance. This output can be measured with either a Foley catheter or a urine-measuring device in the commode.

Most people experience some swelling from the fluid shifts after surgery. This can put additional strain on the heart. The swelling reaches a peak on the third day and then gradually improves, particularly as you begin walking and exercising in general.

Finally, the short-term use of oxygen may also be helpful to prevent cardiac problems following the operation. Your physician should make oxygen available if you are showing signs of cardiac stress in the postoperative period. Recent research indicates that beta-blockers used during your surgery and hospitalization can markedly decrease your risk of death from heart problems linked to the surgery itself. Many patients who could benefit from beta-blocker therapy—notably those with hypertension, angina, or post-myocardial infarction—are not receiving these drugs. If you have heart disease or risk factors for heart disease, your doctor or anesthesiologist may consider starting you on this type of medication.

2. Bleeding and clotting imbalances. With each surgery there needs to be a delicate balance of bleeding and clotting. The body knows that only so much blood can be lost before vitality and life, too, are lost. Thus, in response to surgery, a series of biochemical reactions occur, causing the blood to become thicker or more viscous. During this *coagulation response*, blood cells and platelets clump together and form clots more easily. This adaptive process, which helps prevent excessive bleeding from a wound, also helps inhibit fibrosis, the formation of scar tissue.

The trouble is, an overly strong coagulation response, or *hypercoagulation*, can increase your risk of *thromboembolism*. This is a potentially deadly blockage of a blood vessel to a vital organ, such as the lung. Major surgery is an important risk factor for thromboembolism, especially in cases of orthopedic surgery (hip and knee arthroplasty) and cancer-related surgery.* Elderly and overweight people are even more at risk of developing this complication.

The use of low-molecular-weight heparins and other blood-thinning drugs can be very effective in preventing and treating thromboembolism. (If these anticoagulant drugs fail to reverse the thromboembolism, then a surgery known as thromboembolectomy will be needed.) The problem is not whether or not these anticoagulant drugs work, but that taking them soon after surgery can greatly increase your risk of excessive bleeding. Here's a fairly common scenario to help illustrate this point. Let's say you're an elderly patient and you've been taking anticoagulants for months or even years to prevent heart disease. If your surgeon wants you to temporarily stop taking the anticoagulant, you might suddenly be at increased risk of thromboembolism.[11]

Please note that you generally can undergo dental procedures, arthrocentesis, cataract surgery, and diagnostic endoscopy without changing your anticoagulation regimen.[12] Many types of dermatologic surgery allow you to continue with the regimen as well.[13] For other surgeries, however, your surgeon will probably need to discontinue the blood-thinning drugs temporarily, with aggressive postoperative care and frequent monitoring. Lastly, you may require ongoing warfarin treatment if you have atrial fibrillation, a mechanical heart valve, or a history of venous thromboembolism.

Whether your physician wants to continue with a particular blood-thinning drug such as heparin around the time of surgery will be a highly individualized decision. *Do not make any changes in your anticoagulant regimen on your own; always consult with your physician first.*

For high-risk procedures, your surgeon may recommend *pneumatic compression* stockings and booties. This specialized, therapeutic footwear provides a gentle massage and promotes normal blood flow during and after surgery. As a general rule, the more quickly you can become mobile after your surgery, the less likely you are to "throw a clot," to use the medical jargon. Early walking with as-

---

*We use the term thromboembolism for simplicity's sake. To be more specific, the postoperative complication of interest here is not arterial thromboembolism but *venous thromboembolism,* a term encompassing deep vein thrombosis and pulmonary embolism.

sistance, as soon as possible after surgery (with your physician's permission), can greatly reduce risks of forming a blood clot. Even gentle flexing of the foot and calves while in bed can improve circulation. Gentle massage, with soft strokes up the legs and arms toward the heart, can be done for those who must stay at bed rest. A physical therapist may be helpful if you expect to be bedridden for a more prolonged period.

—Bleeding Risks, Platelets, and Blood-Thinning Drugs and Supplements—

Obviously after your tissues have been cut it is crucial to have the resources in place to stop the bleeding. When these resources are compromised, your blood might not clot well, causing you to lose too much blood. Platelets are one of the key indicators of this clotting ability.

Platelets are disk-shaped particles in the blood that are needed to form blood clots in order to control bleeding and bruising. Low numbers of platelets in your blood indicate a propensity to bleed in an out-of-control manner. In general, if your platelet count is under 20,000 per cubic millimeter of blood, you have a very high risk of spontaneous bleeding.[14] Surgery should be avoided if this is the case. (This condition, known as *thrombocytopenia,* can be controlled by administering certain cytokines or by removing the spleen.)

If your platelet count is between 20,000 and 100,000, you will not have spontaneous bleeding but you do run the risk of excessive bleeding problems—namely, either hemorrhage or wound hematoma—following your surgery. The normal, healthy platelet range is 150,000 to 300,000 per millimeter of blood.

People who have low platelet counts (say, below 80,000) should generally avoid taking powerful anticoagulant drugs such as aspirin, ibuprofen, and warfarin (Coumadin). Certain supplements, namely the ones we've listed in Table 6.2, can amplify a tendency to bleed easily. Keep in mind that the risk would be amplified if you're also taking blood-thinning medications on the same day or within a span of a few days.

Table 6.2. Natural Products That Increase Bleeding: Avoid Taking before Surgery

Botanicals	**Herbs with platelet-inhibiting properties:** garlic, onion, ginkgo, ginseng, feverfew, green tea, ginger, bromelain, clove, turmeric (curcumin)
	Herbs containing coumadin: angelica root, anise, arnica flower, celery, chamomile, fenugreek, horse chestnut, licorice root, lovage root, parsley, passionflower, red clover, sweet clover
	Herbs containing salicylates: meadowsweet, poplar, willow bark
	Other: Bilberry (and other anthocyanidin-containing herbs)
Nutritional supplements*	Vitamin C (in excess of 2 g/day)
	Vitamin E (in excess of 800 IU/day)
	Fish oil and other omega-3 supplements (in excess of 1 g/day)

*The nutritional supplements (as well as most of the herbals) are generally only a problem when taken at high doses or in combination with blood-thinning medications. This assumes, however, that you are not in a high-risk group for bleeding or hemorrhage (e.g., uncontrolled high blood pressure).

Among the most commonly used blood-thinning supplements are ginseng, garlic, ginkgo biloba, vitamin E, vitamin C, and fish oil. At least in theory, these supplements *can* promote blood thinning and therefore increase your risk of excessive bleeding. Nonetheless, since the effects of most of the botanicals listed in the chart have not been well studied in humans, their true blood-thinning impacts remain a matter of speculation. A recent randomized study found that ginkgo and ginger at recommended doses do not adversely affect clotting status or the activity of warfarin, at least not in healthy people.[15] Moreover, even though ginseng has blood-thinning effects, it was recently shown to *reduce* the blood-thinning effects of warfarin.[16]

Other risk factors for excessive bleeding include uncontrolled high blood pressure, anti-inflammatory drugs (e.g., ibuprofen), medications for gout, and of course blood-thinning drugs such as heparin and warfarin (Coumadin). Even a daily dose of aspirin can increase your risk of internal bleeding.

We recommend against using any blood-thinning supplements in the context of the risk factors above. Also, if you've been taking the blood-thinning herbs, avoid them for at least two weeks prior to surgery. With nutrients, the guidelines are more relaxed: one week before surgery is probably more than enough time, and then only if you've been using them in very high doses. As a general rule of thumb, keep your dosages of vitamins C and E moderate, as per our guidelines in above. You should stop supplementing with fish oil a week before the operation—hopefully your body will have enough stored up to provide the protection you need afterward. If you've taken more than two grams of fish oil daily for several weeks, then stop taking fish oil two weeks before surgery.*

Whereas some people bleed too easily, others develop clots too easily (thrombosis)—a tendency that's inherited or may be

————

*If you take Coumadin or other blood-thinning medications or suspect a blood-clotting problem, your physician will want to evaluate you periodically with a blood test called the PT-INR (Prothrombin-International Normalized Ratio). Your doctor will know how to interpret the test results, which will indicate your risk level as well as how well the medications are working. (PT time is a measure of bleeding time and therefore reflects your coagulation status. A high INR means freer-flowing blood and thus a higher risk of dangerous bleeding during and after the surgery.) Remember that some natural agents can make these medicines either more or less strong. Ask your doctor before taking a new medicine, and let him or her know about the dietary supplements you've recently taken.

related to having a prosthetic device.* This can be a problem, since excessive clotting can impede the healing process and also lead to vascular problems. If you find yourself in this category, your doctor may recommend blood-thinning medications after surgery to ward off the excessive clotting response. Other causes for excess clotting include prolonged immobility or abdominal, pelvic, and cancer surgeries. Your surgeon may suggest the use of preventive therapies and medications if you are at high risk for thrombosis. Ideally, your doctor or caregiver will be well-versed in the potential for negative interactions and can advise you appropriately.

_____

*Most of the time, the inherited tendency to increased clotting manifests as a malfunctioning of protein C. This condition is called "APC resistance" or "factor V Leiden." Others do not produce enough antithrombin III, or the antithrombin III they produce does not function well.

Obesity or excessive weight also increases the risk of thromboembolism, as does a dietary history high in saturated fat. A high-fiber, low-fat diet accompanied by omega-3 supplementation prior to surgery will tend to reduce this risk, but be sure to stop taking your omega-3 supplement one week before surgery or if you're on blood-thinning medication. These strategies are highly recommended both before and after surgery if your physician considers you to be at high risk for developing thromboembolism down the road.

Mind-body strategies also play a role in the control of excessive bleeding. You may use hypnosis or self-hypnosis and include the suggestion that bleeding will be minimal and that your circulation will return to normal rapidly. These strategies may reinforce others you're using, such as avoiding high doses of garlic and blood-thinning supplements and medications, to help lower the risk of uncontrolled bleeding.

3. Decreased lung function. Soon after surgery, your lung function can become compromised because of chronic pain, abnormal functioning of the diaphragm (due to cutting into the abdominal area), and increased tension in the abdominal and chest (intercostal) muscles during exhalation. The possible consequences of this *pulmonary dysfunction* are as follows: (1) low blood oxygen levels (*hypoxemia*); (2) a complete or partial collapse of the lung (*atelectasis*); (3) pneumonia; and (4) respiratory failure. Remember that low oxygen levels alone can significantly impede healing, so it's important to prevent and treat this problem as soon as possible.

If you're undergoing either thoracic or upper abdominal surgery, you'll have an increased risk of developing problems with lung function. Others who have a high risk of these and related complications include smokers, the obese, the elderly, people suffering from severe pain, and those with underlying pulmonary disease. You can limit these risks through weight loss, avoiding tobacco smoke, and enhancing your lung function with inhalers (if deemed medically appropriate).

Cardiorespiratory fitness training is the best way to strengthen lung function before and after surgery. If you're in one of the high-risk groups we just mentioned, then consider working with an exercise physiologist or physical therapist who can help you rebuild lung function. Follow our nutritional guidelines in chapter 4. Avoid all mucus-promoting foods such as dairy products, white flour products, sugar, artificial sweeteners, fried foods, saturated fats, sulfites, and other food additives.

To further strengthen the lungs, some health practitioners recommend taking various lung-supporting herbs, such as mugwort, mullein, hyssop, and elecampane. European physicians tend to use these herbs much more often due to a wider acceptance of herbal medicine in Germany, France, and other European countries. Unfortunately, the scientific support for postoperative use of these agents is very scant. Check with your local naturopath or herbalist to determine the proper dosages and timing for use of these herbs.

In order to measure your lung function, your surgeon may recommend the use of an *incentive spirometer* after your operation. This handheld device allows you to track how deeply and fully you are breathing. Using this several times an hour while you are awake during the first few days after surgery can limit many pulmonary complications.

4. Gastrointestinal problems: postoperative nausea, vomiting, and ileus. After surgery, many people experience one or more of three bothersome digestive problems: nausea, vomiting, and a disturbing gut problem called *ileus*. The latter condition usually involves a kind of paralysis of the small intestines (though the colon can also be involved). In the absence of muscular contractions in the intestines, food and wastes do not move easily along the digestive tract, and this can result in cramping, indigestion, constipation, and ultimately, intestinal obstruction. Narcotic pain medications and immobility tend to slow down bowel function and may contribute to the problem. The body's inflammatory pathways seem to be involved in all three aspects of gastrointestinal discord.

Among the more effective ways to control postoperative nausea and vomiting, or PONV, is to use acupuncture both before and after surgery. A meta-analysis of 26 clinical trials concluded that acupuncture was effective in reducing nausea by 28 percent, vomiting by 29 percent, and the need for nausea-countering drugs by 24 percent.[17] Another controlled trial found that women having an abdominal hysterectomy were 38 percent less likely to vomit after their surgery if they received auricular (ear) acupuncture treatments, compared to women who received no acupuncture.[18] Some women undergoing surgery for breast cancer respond very well to acupuncture treatment for PONV.[19]

Incidentally, one of the main types of acupuncture used in these studies involved stimulation of the P6 acupoint (called *Neigun*) on the wrist. In one double-blind, randomized, placebo-controlled study, children undergoing surgery for strabismus (an eye problem) received P6 acupuncture with a low-level laser.[20] Laser stimulation of the P6 acupoint was done 15 minutes before anesthesia and then 15 minutes after arriving in the recovery room. The incidence of vomiting was an impressive 60 percent lower in the laser-acupuncture group than in the placebo group. The efficacy of P6 acupuncture for PONV prevention and relief is, in many surgical situations, similar to commonly used antiemetic drugs.[21] More recently, laser acupuncture was significantly more effective than an antiemetic drug in preventing PONV in children undergoing other types of surgery—hernia repair, circumcision, or orchidopexy.[22]

The use of *acupressure,* applying specific pressure to the P6 acupoint, is also very effective in reducing PONV, according to three controlled trials of women undergoing various kinds of elective gynecological surgery.[23] This point is located 3 cm from the crease at the bottom of the palm, between the tendons of the forearm. Gentle firm massage of this point with manual pressure or with wristbands can be used. The acupressure wristbands can be worn during surgery as well. Acupressure using a different acupoint (K-K9) may help reduce PONV in children.[24] This is a Korean acupressure point located on the middle bone of the ring fingers (palm side). Massaging this point with manual pressure or placement of an acupressure disk for 30 minutes before anesthesia can be beneficial. It has also been shown to improve bowel function after surgery.[25] This is a powerful bodywork technique that could be taught to nurses so that people of all ages would suffer less after surgery.

Nausea and vomiting may affect as many as 8 in every 10 patients who undergo outpatient surgery. In some cases, this can last for up to 5 days after surgery. Drinking ginger tea has been helpful in relieving PONV, though its effects are less well documented than those of acupuncture.[26] Given that PONV is one of the most common causes of hospital readmission after surgery, we feel strongly that acupuncture and acupressure deserve far more serious attention as nonpharmacological solutions. Using either acupuncture or acupressure, it has been estimated that 20 to 25 percent of adults would not experience early PONV.[27]

What's the best way to get acupuncture or acupressure treatments? First, ask your surgeon if your hospital has an acupuncturist on staff. Otherwise, look for a licensed practitioner in your area who can treat you before you have surgery and after you're discharged from the hospital—preferably someone who has experience working with surgical patients.

Other traditional approaches that may be helpful in combating PONV include hypnosis and aromatherapy massage. The essential oils most commonly used for nausea include coriander, lavender, ginger, and fennel. You can put an aromatherapy device in your bedroom or anywhere in your house to provide these aromas throughout the day.

To encourage a return to normal bowel functioning and elimination of PONV, several other strategies are very important. Try to get walking or moving as soon as possible. Second, consider hypnosis, which has been shown to help prevent nausea and vomiting. In a controlled study of breast cancer patients undergoing surgery, those who received hypnosis during the week prior to surgery had about 30 percent less vomiting and nausea and needed less painkilling medication after their operation.[28] This makes sense, given that so much of the reaction to food is influenced by your psyche. Finally, in many cases, osteopathic manipulative therapy can help restore normal function to the digestive system and will reinforce the mind-body approaches mentioned above (see the story of Mr. Menendez).

Mr. Menendez was a sixty-two-year-old man who came to see me after having bypass surgery to improve circulation in his legs. He had very poor circulation because of diabetes. He came to me because his recent operation had triggered several problems. The pain in his upper back and arthritic neck was worse because of the difficult neck position during the surgery and stiffness from the period of inactivity following the surgery. He also had daily stomach and intestinal upset that was not relieved by medications for excess stomach acid. There were many foods he could not eat that had given him no problem before the surgery. He was especially upset because he could not eat the spicy Mexican foods he had loved since childhood.

On my first visit with Mr. Menendez, I offered him a head-to-toe osteopathic treatment to restore normal movement in all parts of his body that I had found to be restricted. At his next visit, he reported to me that he could eat all his favorite foods again and his digestive upset was gone. Over several subsequent visits, his back and neck pain melted away. He still had several major medical issues to deal with, but the discomfort from his surgery had been relieved in the course of helping his body move better.

—TMM

Finally, introduce food sooner rather than later. In the past, surgical patients were advised to consume nothing through the mouth for several days after major abdominal surgery. Recent research indicates, however, that starting to eat the next day encourages healthy digestion. You will likely be started on clear liquids first followed by digestible, "soft" solid foods. Once you have shown that you can tolerate solid foods, you may want to have some nutritious home cooked meals brought in to you. In any case, it's important to attend to your food needs *before* thinking about your supplement options.

Some supplements that aid in restoring healthy digestion include glutamine and aloe vera (see Table 6.3, page 161). Also, assuming you received antibiotics during surgery, the use of probiotic supplements like L-acidophilus for a week after surgery will replenish the normal healthy bacteria in your intestines. For our surgical patients, we often recommend a fiber supplement that is glutamine-enriched and contains aloe and probiotics. They can add a scoop to the Power Healing Drink in the first few weeks after they begin eating regular food. We've noticed a sharp decrease in constipation and bloating since patients have begun using this supplement. Keep in mind that while many whey proteins already contain glutamine, additional glutamine (5 to 10 g per day) may be needed to restore healthy intestinal function.

5. Postoperative cognitive dysfunction. The fifth outcome associated with surgical stress is also one of the most distressing: reduced cognitive function. Varying degrees of cloudy thinking, memory loss, and other expressions of cognitive dysfunction seem to affect everyone during the postoperative period, and much of this may be traced to the use of anesthesia.[29] People over age sixty are particularly susceptible to this problem and it can persist from one week to three months after the surgery.[30] Elderly people are at risk of cognitive dysfunction even after relatively minor surgery, as long as anesthesia is used.[31]

A large percentage of people who undergo coronary bypass surgery may develop cognitive deficits such as short-term memory loss, psychomotor problems (for example, poor reflexes), and "executive dysfunction," a broad term that encompasses problems with higher order thinking, such as problem solving, planning, and developing and implementing strategies.[32] In some cases, the problems may be traced to direct surgical damage to specific nerves, while other cases may be related to the duration of anesthesia or to the stress chemistry evoked by the surgery.

Many diabetic patients experience a decrease in their cognitive ability after undergoing coronary artery bypass surgery. In a recent study of 182 patients, the following risk factors for cognitive dysfunction were found: old age (50 percent increased risk); hypertension (80 percent increased risk); diabetic retinopathy (30 percent increased risk); atherosclerosis of the ascending aorta (50 percent increased risk); poor glucose control (90 percent increased risk); and insulin therapy (200 percent increased risk). All of these factors were associated with cognitive impairment six months after the surgery.[33]

In general, the more dramatic or invasive the surgery, the greater the likelihood that you will experience some lapse in cognitive ability after the operation.[34] The type of anesthesia used may also have an impact. For example, a recent study found that propofol and sevoflurane anesthesia resulted in more postoperative cognitive dysfunction among the elderly.[35] Some researchers have suggested that using neuraxial (spinal, epidural) anesthesia during surgery may decrease postoperative cognitive dysfunction when compared with general anesthesia, though this view remains controversial.[36]

To safeguard cognitive functioning, you might consider the use of acupuncture in place of anesthesia; we discuss this in chapter 8, "Holistic Support for Specific Surgical Scenarios." Several other strategies can be used to support your psyche and enhance your overall well-being after surgery:

- Bring a list of phone numbers you might need and paper and pencil to have by your bed to write down questions for your doctors and staff.

- Pack favorite books and photos, which may help orient you after surgery.

- Keep glasses and hearing aids within reach.

- Have a family member or supportive friend stay with you in the hospital.

- Have an inexpensive clock radio put at the hospital bedside with music, the time, and news to help you stay grounded in time and place. Older patients, especially, might benefit from this.

In addition, there are several supplements that can help bolster cognitive ability and keep you in a clearer frame of mind. These include the following:

- *Ginkgo biloba.* This herb may enhance cerebral circulation and overall brain functioning. Numerous well-controlled clinical studies in Europe and the U.S. have demonstrated that ginkgo has favorable effects in people with memory disorders, dementia, and cerebral impairment due to inadequate blood flow (ischemia); improvement has been found in terms of memory, attention, alertness, vigilance, arousal, and mental fluidity.[37]

People over age fifty may be more likely to show cognitive improvements after taking ginkgo biloba.[38] Though research has not been conducted on the impact of ginkgo on postoperative cognitive dysfunction, this herb is safe enough to try on a precautionary basis. The recommended dosage is 120 to 240 mg per day of the standardized extract, divided into two to three doses. Remember to avoid ginkgo if you're taking blood-thinning medications.

- *Phosphatidylserine.* This is a naturally occurring component of cell membranes that is rapidly absorbed into the brain. Clinical studies demonstrated that taking the supplement improves short-term memory, concentration, and other aspects of cognitive functioning.[39] It has been shown to increase neurotransmitter production as well as the brain's utilization of glucose.[40] Phosphatidylserine also may reduce levels of the stress hormone cortisol, which may explain its antidepressant or mood-enhancing effects.[41] By compensating for low phosphatidylserine levels in the brain, this natural agent may prevent or even reverse age-related cognitive decline.[42] A daily dose of 300 mg is recommended for the first month; then reduce to 100 to 200 mg per day for your maintenance dose.

- *Omega-3 fatty acids (DHA & EPA).* Omega-3 fatty acids increase nerve cell membrane fluidity and may thereby enhance cognition, memory, and mood.[43] A population-based study in Holland found that low dietary intake of omega-3s was significantly correlated with higher rates of cognitive decline.[44] Controlled clinical trials suggest that omega-3 fatty acids can help prevent emotional distress and can further improve conventional treatments for major depression.[45] In terms of surgery, supplementation with docosahexaenoic acid (DHA), one of the omega-3 fatty acids found in fish oil, may be especially helpful in preventing loss of neurons when blood flow to the brain is temporarily restricted (ischemia).[46] A range of 2 to 5 per day, with food, may be helpful. Avoid high-dose fish oil if you are on blood-thinning medication and one week before surgery.

6. Postoperative depression. Another common aftereffect of major surgery is depression.[47] Depression can be brought on by any number of factors, such as a radical change in body image, loss of physical functioning, or stress hormones that contribute to mood disorders. Depression, anxiety, and post-traumatic stress disorder (PTSD) are common outcomes of cardiac surgery.[48] Women seem to be particularly prone to postoperative depression.[49]

Sometimes the results of surgery are less than ideal, and you may be forced to consider further treatment. This can be overwhelming, especially if the surgery you just experienced was fairly stressful. Thoughts of having to go through additional procedures can trigger waves of fear and depression. These negative feelings and the physiologic responses that accompany them are detrimental to tissue healing and the immune system.

Psychotherapy or group support before and after surgery can help prevent depression after the operation.[50] Improving your immediate environment can also help lift your spirits. Consider the following:

- Flowers, family photos, cards, and personal keepsakes can make a hospital or recovery room warmer and less sterile.

- A portable music player will allow you to listen to your own music or books on tape.

- Magazines, funny or inspiring tapes, or books can help prevent boredom.

- Sacred objects such as medallions or beads, or various religious symbols may provide spiritual and emotional comfort.

- Home-cooked food, when you are eating again may can have a soothing effect.

- Aromatherapy by your bed may ease your negative thoughts. Lavender, lemon balm, chamomile, clary sage, and ylang ylang are good choices. You may want to sample some scents to see what you like or speak to an aromatherapist before surgery.

- Allowing yourself time to heal is crucial. Take a vacation from caring for everyone else and nurture yourself with rest and relaxation. A guilt-free vacation from being in charge of everything can help alleviate anxiety and depression.

In addition, several supplements have been shown to improve mood, stave off depression. Earlier, on pages 153–154, we mentioned omega-3s, phosphatidylserine, and ginkgo biloba—all three of which may not only give you a cognitive boost but lift your spirits as well. Other mood-enhancing supplements include the following:

- **SAM-e.** S-adenosylmethionine (SAM-e) is an amino acid supplement that may also have mood- and cognition-enhancing effects.[51] An oral dose of 400 to 1,600 mg per day is recommended for depression.

- **Saint-John's-wort.** Saint-John's-wort is another herbal antidepressant with good evidence of effectiveness in combating mild, moderate, and severe depression. However, there are concerns about its interactions with antidepressants, narcotics, and other medications. A safe daily dosage is 2 to 4 grams of the dried plant, or 300 to 600 mg per day if a liquid extract is used. If you are on any medication, check with your doctor first before taking Saint-John's-wort.

- **Bacopa.** *Bacopa monniera*, also known as *Brahmi,* is an East Indian herb that has clinically demonstrated antianxiety and memory-enhancing effects.[52] The usual dose of bacopa is 100 mg of the standardized extract, one to three times daily. This herb is increasingly being added to other supplements designed to enhance brain function, such as ginkgo biloba.

- **5HTP**. 5HTP is an amino acid supplement that helps your body make the neurotransmitter serotonin and may provide relief for depression.[53] This is especially recommended for people who are suffering from *both* depression and poor sleep quality, because it boosts the production of melatonin at night.[54] The effective dosage range is between 50 and 300 mg. Higher doses are not recommended.

7. Suppressed immunity. Surgery is almost always followed by a temporary period of weakened or depressed immunity. In some cases, your immune system may be dangerously suppressed due to surgical stress. Depending on your age, overall health, and the nature of the surgery, the immune suppression can last for days, weeks, or even months.[55]

Depressed immunity can have troubling consequences, such as increasing your risk of becoming infected with staphylococci (staph infection, which is common in the hospital environment) or contracting other infections. Such infections increase your risk for wound separation and failed healing. Also, surgical adjuncts like anesthetics and other pharmacologic interventions can further dampen your body's ability to mount an effective immune response against bacteria and other infectious organisms. When the immune suppression is severe and prolonged, it can lead to sepsis or other life-threatening infections.[56] For people who are having tumors removed, the depressed immunity can also set the stage for recurrences or even for new cancers.[57]

Antimicrobial and anticancer agents can be used to treat these problems, of course; however, the worldwide problem of antibiotic resistance should temper our reliance on antibiotics.* A more proactive strategy is to try to prevent these problems from cropping up in the first place—by keeping your immune system strong and helping it recover from the stressful effects of the surgery.

We believe that more attention should be given immediately to enhancing immune competence and to reducing the risks posed by postoperative immune

---

*Each time new antibiotics are introduced, some bacteria will resist the drugs and go on to multiply, creating larger and larger numbers of antibiotic-resistant bacteria over time. According to the FDA, about 70 percent of bacteria that cause infections in hospitals are resistant to at least one of the drugs most commonly used to treat infections. Antibiotic drugs given to food-producing animals can cause microbes to become resistant to drugs used to treat human illness, ultimately making some infections harder to treat. Disease-causing bacteria that have become resistant to antibiotics are a grave public health problem.

suppression. After all, the sooner you recover your immune function, the better your chances are of surviving those life-threatening infections should they arise.[58] Fortunately, there are many things you can do to boost your T cells (lymphocyte blood cells that help fight infection and natural killer cells (NK cells) activity after surgery. Your physician may suggest the use of pharmaceutical immune-enhancing agents, such as interferons, interleukins, and colony-stimulating factors. While these strategies certainly have merit, we encourage all our patients to look to natural methods first, including a low-fat, vegetable-rich diet and various supplements that have been shown to bolster immune function (see Table 6.3).

In terms of supporting people undergoing surgery, one of the best studied of the natural immune enhancers is the amino acid glutamine. Glutamine is the primary fuel for cells that are rapidly dividing, such as immune cells and cells that comprise the intestinal lining.[59] In one study glutamine supplementation in surgical patients resulted in enhanced NK and T-cell functioning, as well as improved survival from infection and better postoperative results in general.[60] Numerous randomized double-blind clinical studies have now shown that when glutamine is taken following elective surgery, the rate of recovery increases, less time is spent in the hospital, and there is a significant drop in postoperative infectious complications.[61]

Glutamine is an example of a nutrient that may become "conditionally essential" during inflammatory conditions such as injury or infection.[62] This means that your body needs more of the amino acid depending on how much it has been stressed by an infection or by an invasive procedure. People who have taken plenty of antibiotics or received treatments that can damage the intestines—abdominal surgery or chemotherapy, for example—can also take higher doses of glutamine. This can exert a profound influence on the digestive system and improve overall health: By speeding up the regeneration of the intestinal mucosa, glutamine reduces the likelihood of bacteria and toxins entering into the bloodstream, and this, in turn, reduces the tendency toward chronic inflammation.[63]

One of our patients had a kidney disease that caused her to lose excessive amounts of protein in her urine. This loss of protein, in turn, interfered with her immune system's functioning. She had surgery to drain an abscess. Her healing was delayed until she began to use high doses of glutamine along with vitamin C and other nutritional supplements.

Arginine, another key amino acid, has also been studied extensively in people exposed to surgical stress. Usually it has been combined with omega-3 fatty acids and dietary nucleotides (the building blocks of DNA) to form "immunonutrition" enteral formulas.* Enteral feeding involves placing a tube through the stomach. Most of the patients who require enteral formulas are critically ill. The usual surgery patient will not require enteral formulas but will eat a regular diet. Nonetheless, we feel that the data from the clinical trials show how important a nutrient it is for immune function.

Patients on regular diets who would like to enhance their immune function may want to add arginine in supplement form, either as capsules or powder (see Table 6.3). This is one of several nutrients that comprise the so-called immunutrition approach. Clinical trials have demonstrated that supplementing with these nutrients results in less chronic inflammation, better immune function, fewer infectious complications, and a faster overall recovery from major surgery.[64] In addition to the immune-boosting effects, it also stimulates the release of growth hormone; however, arginine should be avoided by critically ill individuals with preexisting severe sepsis (the presence of disease-causing organisms or their toxins in the blood or tissues) due to concerns about potential adverse effects; in addition, arginine should generally not be taken by people with cancer, diabetes, arthritis, herpes or shingles.

Based on the pooled results of 26 clinical trials, European researchers offered the following conclusions about the benefits of immunonutrition.

- Patients receiving immunonutrition showed a 74 percent reduction in the rate of infections. The incidence of pneumonia and bacteremia dropped by 46 and 55 percent, respectively.

---

* The term *enteral* refers to those nutritional preparations that are provided through a tube in the stomach; such preparations are for people who cannot take food through the mouth yet still have an intact digestive system.

- There was a reduced dependency on mechanical ventilation, with the immunonutrition patients using it an average of about 2.25 days less than other patients.

- Time spent in the intensive care unit, or ICU, was reduced by nearly 2 days on average, while the average time spent in the hospital was reduced by nearly 3.5 days.[65]

Arginine, glutamine, and other supplements we list in Table 6.3 are excellent choices following surgery because they have been shown to enhance immune function in various ways. Nonetheless, be aware of potential side effects, dosage issues, and interactions with medications. Use the table as a starting point in your education about the natural immune stimulants that have the most research behind them. It would be a good idea to check with your integrative medical practitioner about possible adverse reactions and interactions with medications you may be taking before starting.

If you do experience any signs of infection after your surgery—fever, redness around the wound, drainage of yellow fluid, bad odor, or wound opening—be sure to contact your doctor immediately. Saline is the best fluid to clean any wound (hydrogen peroxide and iodine-based solutions inhibit healing). With proper antibiotics and wound cleaning, most wounds can be safely reclosed within 4 days and healing restored. For severe infections or deep wounds in heavy patients, many surgeons will use a vacuum drain that a home health nurse can change to further speed healing after an infection.

ᕫ Dealing with Surgical Pain the Holistic Way

"When will I be free of pain?" People who have just undergone surgery often ask this question, and for good reason. Pain is a universal experience and a common concern for anyone facing surgery. Eight out of every 10 surgical patients will have pain after their procedure.[66] Managing that pain is almost as much art as it is science, which is why anesthesiology, the study of pain, is a whole medical specialty unto itself. Thanks to recent advances in medicine, you can now obtain excellent pain relief with far fewer adverse effects than in the past.

Table 6.3. Immune-Enhancing Supplements to Consider after Surgery

IMMUNE ENHANCER	BENEFITS AND PRACTICAL CONSIDERATIONS (TO BE USED FROM ONE TO THREE MONTHS AFTER SURGERY)*
Glutamine	Recommended dose is 800 mg per day, though doses ranging from 5,000 to 20,000 mg have been used in severe cases.
Arginine	Recommended dosage range is 15 to 20 g per day for one week before and after major surgery.
Omega-3 fatty acids	3 to 5 g per day for the first month after surgery (though ideally this should start before surgery; see chapter 4).
Vitamin C	1 to 4 g per day, in divided doses (500 mg) spread out over the course of the day, in buffered, time-release capsule form, with bioflavonoids.
Mushrooms (maitake, reishi, shitake, cordyceps, and coriolus)	Many preparations available; use only standardized extracts, and take as directed on the label.
Echinacea	1 g of dried root three times a day, or as a tea consisting of 1 g of dried root in a pint of boiling water three times a day.
Ginseng (American and Asian)	200 to 600 mg per day as capsules, or one cup of tea three times a day. A ginseng-free period of 1 to 2 weeks is recommended every 4 to 6 weeks.
Aloe vera	100 to 200 mg of the juice in the morning and evening, orally; additional amounts may be taken as long as the anthraquinones (laxative components) have been removed.

*If laboratory tests indicate that you have severe immune suppression, consider taking these agents in the higher level of the range, but again only under expert supervision. The omega-3 fatty acids can suppress immune function at high levels, so care must be exercised when adjusting dosages.

—Harnessing Life Energy to Bolster Your Immune Defenses—

Acupuncture and acupressure points can be used to promote health and support the immune system. The concept of boosting Chi, or life force, is one that does not have a good equivalent in Western medicine. Here's a short acupressure series that can be done by yourself to boost your immune function. A licensed acupuncturist or acupressure practitioner (also called shiatsu) can provide a more individualized treatment for you if you feel you would benefit from a more tailored approach.

This series can be done sitting or lying down with a tennis ball applied to the points. Altogether it will take about 5 to 10 minutes and can be performed daily. Be sure to take slow deep breaths while massaging the points.

Start with B36, the so-called Bearing Support point. To locate this point, feel for the top of the shoulder blade and move along it until you find the tip near the spine—the point lies just off the tip near the spine. Apply firm pressure for one minute to each side. Pressure from a tennis ball can also work. To use a tennis ball lie on your back on the floor and place a tennis ball under your upper back between your spine and shoulder blade; after one minute move it to the other side.

Next, try to locate the Sea of Vitality points (B23 and B47). Sit forward on your chair for the next points. Place the backs of your hands against your lower back. Rub up and down for one minute, creating some warmth in the area. You can also apply warm heat with a heating pad to these points or use pressure from a tennis ball. To use a tennis ball lie on your back on the floor and place a tennis ball under your lower back behind your belly button 1.5 cm to the side of the spine. After a minute, move it to the other side.

Finish with firm gentle pressure for one minute to CV 17, the Sea of Tranquility, point: Place your palms together, place the back of your thumbs firmly against your breastbone at the level of your heart. Keep your eyes closed and concentrate on breathing slow, even, deep breaths into your heart for one minute.

Pain has two central components. The first is the organic component caused by your nerves sensing damage to the tissue. The second is the psychological aspect. This includes fear, memories of pain, cultural and family beliefs and responses to pain, and the expectation of relief. This psychological response to pain—and in particular the meaning we ascribe to pain—tends to intensify the suffering we experience. A truly holistic approach to pain calls for addressing both issues.

Managing your pain as best as you possibly can is essential to how well you heal following surgery. Why would this be the case? The hormonal and nervous system responses to pain tend to intensify the surgical stress response. For this reason, pain can further delay the return to normal functioning.[67] Postoperative pain is among the leading causes of readmission to a same-day surgical unit. In this section, we discuss some of the ways you can cope with pain from the standpoint of integrative medicine.

Our first bit of practical advice for those dealing with the pain of surgery is simply this: relax. There are many ways to obtain pain relief, and medications are an excellent first option. Local anesthetics, injected into the area around the incision, have proved to be beneficial in minor surgeries. Peripheral nerve blocks work well in orthopedic surgeries, and a continuous peripheral nerve blockade has proved to be safe and effective if you're being treated on an outpatient basis.

Epidural anesthesia, also known as epidural block, is an effective way to provide pain relief in many major surgery situations. Epidural anesthesia may be used as an alternate for or in conjunction with general anesthesia and can be continued, if needed, after the operation for continued excellent pain control. This procedure involves the injection of pain medication into the space surrounding the spinal cord, partially numbing the abdomen and lower body. The epidural strategy (versus general anesthesia) diminishes the harmful effects of surgical stress and reduces the need for oral painkilling medications—and also complements the effects of those medications.[68] Specifically, by blocking nerve signals to and from the spinal cord, epidural anesthesia can help preserve normal lung function, get your digestive system working again, and lower your risk of pneumonia, thromboembolism, and cardiac complications.[69]

One of the best strategies for pain numbing after surgery is an analgesia intravenous pump that you control yourself. This so-called patient-controlled analgesia, or PCA, involves a computerized device that gives you a specific dose of painkilling medication with the push of a button, whenever you feel that you need it. The button is located beside your bed, within easy reach. This means you do not have to call for a nurse to relieve pain or discomfort. Although the PCA pump provides potent painkilling medication, it is preprogrammed by your anesthesiologist to prevent any chance of overdose. And contrary to popular beliefs, the risk of addiction is extremely low—very close to zero—as is the case with other postoperative pain medications.[70] An anti-inflammatory medicine may be added to the mix to reduce the amount of narcotic you use. Once you can eat again, you will be switched to an oral pain medication.

These oral medications can and almost always should be taken on a regular schedule rather then waiting for the pain to return and get unbearable. You may be given an oral medication to take every 3 or 4 hours during the first few days after surgery or after your hospital discharge. Many of the oral or injected analgesics will begin to take effect within 20 minutes, reaching their peak effectiveness within an hour. They typically continue to provide relief for about 3 to 4 hours, though will become less effective toward the third hour. Being aware of this "peak and valley" effect will help you to deal better with the pain before it returns. Finding distracting activities can be helpful in the interim, but be ready to remedicate yourself as needed. For more severe pain, your doctor may give you a pain medication that lasts for 6 to 12 hours.

If you're discharged from the hospital the same day as your surgery, your doctor may recommend a long-acting local anesthetic to reduce pain for the first evening at home. Then a combination of oral narcotics and anti-inflammatory agents should provide excellent relief.

Be aware that most narcotics can cause some constipation. Plan to use a stool softener like colace while you are taking narcotics such as hydrocodone, oxycodone, codeine, and morphine. Another side effect is the drug-induced suppression of natural killer cell activity and other immune functions. This has been known since the late 1800s, when scientists administered morphine to guinea pigs and observed an elevated rate of bacterial infections.[71] For people with cancer, the risk of metastases may also increase with morphine use. These are just some additional reasons why you don't want to be on these pain medications for very long, and why alternatives such as acupuncture have so much value.

Acupuncture is, in fact, a very effective way to control pain in people undergoing surgery.[72] Research shows that acupuncture and electroacupuncture can substantially reduce the need for pain-killing medication following surgery.[73] The use of *preoperative* acupuncture also may have a pain-relieving effect following the surgery.[74] Acupuncture seems to accomplish this feat by stimulating the body's built-in pain-relieving mechanisms such as the production of endorphins and other natural opioids.[75] Given the inherent side effects and postoperative complications associated with many analgesic drugs, acupuncture should be considered a valuable addition to any postoperative treatment plan—even though it tends to be less effective than narcotic pain killers.

Acupressure can also be used to reduce pain. One of the most common massage points for pain management is LI4, located in the web of skin between the thumb and index finger on each hand. To find the point, extend your thumb and index finger; the point lies slightly to the finger side on the flesh between the bones of the thumb and index finger. Applying firm pressure or circular rubbing to this point can be a useful adjunct to traditional pain management.

In some cases, postsurgery acupuncture or electroacupuncture may be carried out along side the use of transcutaneous electrical nerve stimulation, or TENS. TENS devices are designed to stimulate a nerve by passing electrical currents through the skin, with pain-relieving results. In a study of women undergoing either total hysterectomy or myomectomy, the use of TENS devices produced pain relief similar to acupuncture, and both were significantly more effective than the placebo or "sham" treatment.[76] Another clinical trial showed that TENS, used in combination with conventional painkillers after abdominal surgery, resulted in a more rapid return to normal walking and a significant postoperative reduction in pain intensity during walking and deep breathing.[77]

We've found that these so-called energetic approaches—acupuncture, acupressure, electroacupuncture, and TENS—often do work very well together or in combination with pain-killing medications and ice treatment.[78] By relying more on these nonpharmacological methods, you can reduce your need for pain medications and thus avoid some of the problems and pitfalls associated with the overuse of these medications.

Osteopathic manipulation, myofascial release, and massage are all forms of bodywork that can diminish pain. These hands-on techniques can be started immediately after the surgery. The practitioner will gently manipulate the tissues, including muscles, joints, and fascia (a type of connective tissue). The improved circulation of blood and lymph and the reduction in muscle spasms can aid in the elimination of pain chemicals (e.g., lactic acid) and toxins from the body, thereby alleviating pain and reestablishing normal movement and breathing.

We've had many patients who chose to combine osteopathic manipulation with massage, electrical stimulation, and acupuncture to relieve pain. This use of multiple modalities can markedly reduce the need for narcotics, as well as decrease digestive upset and increase the ease with which you can move and breathe. Several of our patients have shown dramatic improvements with a combination of osteopathic manipulation, injections of local anesthetics to trigger points, and prolotherapy, an injection therapy that help strengthen loose ligaments. These same modalities also have been helpful in relieving the chronic pain that sometimes occurs when scar tissue develops or wounds do not heal well.

Lastly you may also want to explore the use of hypnosis either as an alternative or as an adjunct to pain medication. With the help of hypnosis, you can change the signals you get from a painful source; you can transform a sharp pain into a tingle, making it much more comfortable to live with. In any case, be sure that you have a plan to deal with the psychological component of pain. Remember that the way you respond to your pain psychologically can influence the intensity of the pain itself. Discuss your fears, beliefs, and expectations with your surgeon and anesthesiologist. Try to identify a relaxation technique that works well for you if you begin to feel anxious (see chapter 5). By laying out a comprehensive plan ahead of time, you may find that your postoperative recovery ends up being a very comfortable experience and that you will greatly reduce the amount of time you spend in the hospital or on pain medication.[79]

RECOVERY THROUGH TOUCH

Betty Ross, a pleasant seventy-three-year-old woman, had undergone abdominal surgery for colon cancer. Older people have an increased frequency of undesirable results and complications following this type of surgery. Compared to younger patients, they're also more likely to enter the operation with advanced-stage cancer and to require emergency surgery.

The first night after surgery, Betty felt a pain in her chest and rang up the nurse, who notified the doctor on call, and he promptly went to check on her. His first concern was that she might be at risk of a heart attack, but subsequent EKG testing and cardiac enzyme panels indicated no serious problems with her heart. Betty again called the nurse about chest pain the following night. The doctor on call ordered a full cardiac evaluation of her heart function, and again the tests turned up negative. On her third night after surgery, Mrs. Ross was still experiencing pain and discomfort, and it had become very difficult for her to sleep.

At this point, I was the doctor on call who was summoned to her bedside. Once again, EKG testing showed nothing out of the ordinary, and her heart and lungs sounded completely normal on stethoscope exam. My assessment of her spine, ribs, and chest revealed tenderness and restricted breathing, as well as decreased mobility. Lying in a hospital bed, many patients can become stiff and rigid from lack of movement, and Betty's long surgery under anesthesia had no doubt exacerbated the stiffness. These factors, together with the anxiety she was experiencing about her imminent chemotherapy treatments, had led to a severe malfunctioning of the muscles in her chest wall.

After my exam, I told Betty what I had found and explained her situation from the osteopathic perspective. With her consent, I then performed gentle manipulation of her thoracic spine, rib cage, and diaphragm for about fifteen minutes, and this brought her a great deal of relief. She began to breathe more freely, color returned to her face, and she no longer felt the uncomfortable constriction around her upper torso. I feel certain that the improvement was not only due to realigning her ribs and spine, but also to the profound healing effect that compassionate touch can have.

So often in the world of high-tech medicine, patients interact with gadgets and machines rather than human beings. Hands-on approaches such as massage, osteopathic manipulation, and acupressure can have a tremendous therapeutic impact, in part, simply because of the human connection—the healing wonders of touch. That night, and all the remaining nights in the hospital, Mrs. Ross had a good night's sleep. Everyone else including the nurses and on-call physicians could all breathe easier too.

All of us have an inner ability to heal ourselves. As a health care practitioner, I know that I do not actually heal people: I merely encourage my patient's inner healer to come forth. I help my patients integrate their body and emotions with their own inner healer. This integration of mind, body, and spirit is the true basis of good medicine.

—TMM

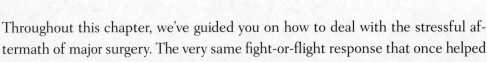

Throughout this chapter, we've guided you on how to deal with the stressful aftermath of major surgery. The very same fight-or-flight response that once helped us deal with the threat of wild beasts actually works against us in the context of modern-day surgery. In general, the bigger and deeper the incision, the greater the stress response will be—and the more suppressed and lethargic your repair processes will be as well. As a consequence, your recovery time will be substantially prolonged, especially if you're over age forty and not exactly in tip-top physical condition.

Nevertheless, with the right program you can greatly temper the stress response and instead promote a strong healing response. The holistic approach we've outlined in this chapter can help you avoid complications, with each of your organ systems functioning smoothly. This program, which we will expand on in the next chapter, will help you rapidly return to good health. With the right combination of therapies, relaxation techniques, nutrition, and rest, you will soon be able to eat normally, move around without pain, think clearly, and feel upbeat about your recovery.

7

Rapid Repair for the Postoperative Period

A time to heal, a time to break down,
and a time to build up . . .

—PROVERBS

Larry Johnson was a seventy-three-year-old wiry tobacco farmer when his daughter-in-law brought him to see me. Four years earlier he had fallen off his farm truck and injured two disks in his lower back. Arthritis and degenerative changes had cropped up in several locations along his spine. Despite having had two spinal surgeries, Larry still had persistent pain in his right lower back that radiated down to the top of his pelvis. On most days he rated his pain as 6 to 7 on a scale from one to 10, but some days it was as bad as 9 or even 10. The pain soon became so severe that he could no longer work his farm or go hunting or fishing with his friends. At that point, he became dependent on his son's family for his food, transportation, and shelter.

Larry and I reviewed his diet and lifestyle. He had always been a meat-and-potatoes guy. But his number one vice was cigarettes: he had smoked two packs a day his whole life and told me bluntly, "I'm not going to quit now." He was nearly as reluctant to cut back on his habit of drinking at least a few beers a day.

My examination revealed that Larry had developed a severe strain in the *connective tissue, muscles, and ligaments that went from his lower back to his pelvis. His ligaments had not healed properly. We talked about what it would take to support his healing process. I felt that even starting after his surgeries there was still a lot we could do to accelerate his recovery and perhaps even give him a new lease on life.*

First we started with his nutrition. I prescribed fish oil, a good multivitamin, and an herbal anti-inflammatory (Itis-Care from Narula Research). His daughter-in-law agreed to help him get more vegetables into his daily diet and to cut back his intake of saturated fats and refined foods. Larry said he was willing to go along with these changes if it would help him return more quickly to his former activity levels. He also agreed to drink only one or two beers a day. I suggested that cutting back on the cigarettes would further bolster his healing, but that was one change he frankly told me he could not make.

Over several months, I saw Mr. Johnson for several body-centered therapies. I did osteopathic manipulation to his strained muscles and connective tissue. For his poorly healed ligaments, I gave him a series of prolotherapy injections (injection of solutions that restimulate healing and strengthen tissues). Over several weeks, as the damaged ligament in his lower back (iliolumbar) started to heal, the strain around and across from it also resolved. During the hands-on sessions, he started to speak to me about how angry he had become about what had happened to his land. I encouraged him to give vent to the anger and taught him breathing techniques to help him prevent the anger from getting bottled up in tight muscles again.

At the end of three months, Larry's daily pain rating had dropped back down to the lowest possible level—most days, he didn't notice any pain whatsoever—and to his delight he was back to fishing and hunting. He even had felt up to taking his grandsons along on his most recent trip. I felt gratified to see how far he had come on his healing journey.

—TMM

So far, we've introduced you to the basics of getting fit for surgery. You've also learned about the essential elements of surgical stress and about natural options for dealing with various postsurgery setbacks. Against that backdrop, let's now consider some of the ways you can use foods and supplements to further fortify your healing foundation and keep you feeling and functioning your best after your operation. If you're coming to this book after already having had surgery, you may be jumping to this chapter before all the rest. That's understandable, but please refer to the earlier chapters, especially chapters 3 and 4, to deepen your appreciation of the powerful impact food can have on your self-healing potential.

Surgical stress drains your body of its nutrient reserves. The increased metabolic demand posed by the stress response means that your cells and tissues need more energy and an increased supply of various vitamins, minerals, proteins, carbohydrates, and fatty acids. Without meeting this increased demand, your body will become depleted of the very nutrients it needs for tissue repair. Surgical stress also has a detrimental effect on appetite and digestion. When your appetite is suppressed and your digestion impaired, it's very easy to become nutritionally depleted. This is precisely the time when you should be ramping up your nutrition to the highest possible level.

Sadly, nutrition is not seen as a high priority in many hospitals, despite the fact that poor nutrition delays recovery, increases the risk of mortality, and boosts the cost of hospitalization.[1] One study found that surgical patients who were poorly nourished spent about 8 days longer in the hospital than their well-nourished counterparts.[2] Clearly, as Hippocrates understood, food and medicine are intimately connected—or at least they should be.

Malnutrition occurs when your nutrient intake isn't enough to meet your requirements.[3] Upon admission to a hospital, 30 to 50 percent of all patients either are or eventually become malnourished.[4] This problem is especially common in the acute-care clinical setting, which is where you find yourself immediately after major surgery. Elderly patients, AIDS and cancer patients, and individuals who have had surgery involving the gastrointestinal system are at the highest risk. Even when a hospital diet is consumed in its entirety, nutritional deficiencies are strikingly common. Consider these findings:

- According to a 1999 study reported in JAMA, many hospitalized elderly patients are undernourished in terms of their overall caloric intake; they are maintained on nutrient intakes (fat, protein, and carbohydrates) way below their estimated caloric needs.[5]

- Patients in a geriatric long-stay care hospital who consumed low-calorie diets were *about 13 times more likely to die in six months* than patients with adequate calorie intakes.[6]

- Even when consuming a 2,000 calorie diet in either the hospital or retirement home, elderly patients often do not consume sufficient quantities of vitamins (in particular, vitamin E and pantothenic acid) and minerals (calcium, zinc, copper, and manganese) to meet recommended levels.[7] Other important deficits affecting elderly patients are a lack of proteins, selenium, and vitamins B_1, B_6, B_{12}, and D.[8]

- In at least seven out of every ten cases, according to a recent report by nutrition researchers at the University of Glasgow (United Kingdom), hospital malnutrition may go unrecognized and therefore unmanaged.[9]

As we showed in earlier chapters, some of the nutrient requirements that are not being met in the hospital setting—notably protein, zinc, and vitamins A and C—are increased as a direct result of the surgery itself. Deficiencies of these and other nutrients can hamper your ability to self-heal.[10] Even when your diet is relatively good, you may need to take additional amounts of these key nutrients immediately after the surgery in order to make sure your tissues repair as well as possible and to shorten your recovery time.[11]

Protein and calories. Simply getting enough protein and calories after your surgery can make a difference in your ability to heal well and avoid complications after the operation. An adequate amount of protein is crucial since all of your body tissues are primarily made of protein. Calories come from carbohydrates and fats and are needed to fuel the repair mechanisms. While major surgery significantly raises your protein and calorie needs, minor surgery should not require any substantial dietary changes. Data from three randomized controlled clinical trials found that taking a protein and energy supplement after hemiarthroplasty (hip fracture surgery) helped reduce infections and other negative outcomes by 48 percent.[12] In other research, undernourished patients who consumed a diet containing 24 percent protein showed a faster resolution of pressure ulcers when compared to patients on a diet containing 14 percent protein.[13] (Pressure ulcers, more commonly known as bedsores, are a wound-healing challenge often faced by people who become bedridden or largely immobilized after surgery. Good nutrition also seems to help *prevent* this problem in the first place.)[14]

Supplemental use of protein powders, liquid proteins, or dietary proteins (egg white, goat's milk, rice protein) can reinforce the effects of a varied, balanced diet. Even if you're required to be on a clear liquid diet following an abdominal surgery, there are now clear liquid protein supplements that you can purchase or obtain from some hospitals. This is especially important if your nutrition was poor before the surgery or you had not been able to eat for several days before the surgery (for example, a long labor before a C-section). Your doctor may want to check a pre-albumin level to see if your protein nutrition is adequate. Once you're eating a regular diet, protein powders such as whey protein and soy protein can be added to the Power Healing Drink.

The normal daily protein requirement for an adult is just over 0.4 grams per pound of body weight, or about 9 grams of protein for every 20 pounds of body weight. This is the amount needed to keep the body from slowly breaking down its own tissues. A better benchmark for maintaining good health, assuming a moderate level of physical activity, would be about 0.6 grams per pound of body weight.

In the first few weeks after major surgery, your daily needs can easily *double*—going up to 1 gram of protein per pound of body weight or even 1.5 grams per pound of body weight.* Nevertheless, because many people will be very sedentary or possibly even bedridden for a while after surgery, we don't recommend that everyone follow this formula to the note. Heavier individuals, in particular, should guard against a simplistic translation from body weight to protein needs. For example, a 200-pound man coming out of surgery should eat about 90 grams of protein per day and no more than 130 grams daily until he is more mobile and begins to engage in exercise.

After you've become more physically active, and depending on the intensity

---

*For those thinking in metric terms, one pound is equivalent to 0.45 kilograms. Thus, a 120-pound woman weighs about 54 kilograms; a 180-pound man weighs about 82 kilograms. The normal daily protein requirement for an adult is 0.8 grams per kilogram of body weight each day, and about twice that amount for people recovering from surgery.

of your exercise routine, your protein intake can shift toward the higher part of the ranges shown in Table 7.1. Keep in mind, though, that protein needs will vary from person to person based upon many different factors. Men tend to need more protein than women, and people with more physically active jobs (e.g., carpentry, construction, farming) require more protein than sedentary people. Protein needs also increase during adolescence, and women have higher protein requirements during pregnancy and breast feeding. Various diseases and medical conditions will further increase the body's protein needs.

The bottom line, though, is that your daily protein intake should also be roughly proportionate to your body size, the severity of your surgery, *and* how much exercise you're getting. A registered dietitian, or RD, can help you figure out how much protein and calorie-rich food is specifically best for you. To find an RD in your area, go to www.eatright.org.

Table 7.1 shows you how your particular body weight translates into your daily protein needs and servings of protein in the weeks following surgery. As you can see, for most adults in the postsurgery phase, a good daily intake means getting three to four servings of protein-rich food a day. That's a solid guideline and can easily be met with the help of fish, legumes, yogurt, whey, and egg whites. For additional ideas on healthy food choices that provide protein, please also refer to Table 4.1 (page 67).

Staying within the higher part of the range of protein consumption for a few weeks after major surgery should not be harmful for most people (the exception being people with kidney problems). Ideally, however, your daily protein intake should not exceed 100 grams per day unless you're exercising daily. The reason for this is that eating more than that amount can lead to protein overload, since the sedentary or inactive body can only handle so much protein. As noted earlier, protein overload can result in such problems as fatigue and weakened immunity, ultimately undermining your efforts to speed up your recovery.

If you do consume extra protein, try to drink plenty of water and engage in exercise that uses the weight-bearing muscles on a daily basis—preferably a combination of weight training and aerobic workouts. This will help your body store some of the protein as muscle and will support better overall fitness.

A very practical question is, how much food corresponds to a serving of protein? The amounts vary, of course, because of the fat content of some high-

Table 7.1. Meeting Your Daily Protein Needs Following Surgery

Body Weight (pounds, kilograms)	Recommended Range of Daily Protein (grams)	Range of Daily Intake for Protein Servings* †
90 pounds (about 40 kg)	40–80 grams	1.5 to 2.5 servings
110 pounds (50 kg)	50–90 grams	2 to 3 servings
130 pounds (60 kg)	60–100 grams	2 to 3.5 servings
155 pounds (70 kg)	70–110 grams	2.5 to 3.5 servings
175 pounds (80 kg)	80–120 grams	2.5 to 4 servings
200 pounds (90 kg)	90–130 grams	3 to 4.5 servings
220 pounds (100 kg)	100–140 grams	3 to 4.5 servings

* People who have recently gone through surgery should eat more servings; however, getting regular exercise is highly recommended for anyone eating over 100 grams per day.

† 1 ounce = 28 grams = 1 serving of protein.

protein foods. But in general, an ounce of lean meat is equivalent to about one serving of protein. Stated more visually, a serving of animal protein the size of a deck of cards is about 3 ounces, or three protein servings. So, for example, a small fish fillet (3 inches × 3 inches) is about 3 ounces, which is equal to about three protein servings. Below are some other examples of how certain high-protein foods translate into a single serving of protein:

- 1 ounce of fish, poultry, wild game, or grass-fed, hormone-free beef
- ¼ cup salmon, lobster, or cottage cheese
- 2 to 3 shrimp, oysters, or scallops
- 1 cup of yogurt
- 1 to 2 scoops of whey protein (depending on quality of supplement)

- 1 egg
- 1 cup well-cooked pinto beans or other beans
- ⅓ chicken breast (or 1 small chicken drumstick)

To further flesh out your options, you may want to refer to Table 7.2, which shows the protein content of various foods in relation to typical serving sizes. This table, coupled with Table 7.1, can also be useful when you're trying to nail down some of the ways you can better meet your protein needs.

Superfoods. Given the serious consequences of some nutritional deficits, it would be helpful for you to follow the nutritional suggestions we laid out in earlier chapters, and to make your physician and nurses aware of your personal desire to have sound nutrition. The Power Healing Drink may be especially helpful in this regard, as it provides concentrated plant-based nutrition as well as whey protein, glutamine, and aloe vera—all are extremely good for your body in this sometimes challenging period immediately following surgery.

Another superfood preparation that may be of value here is a liquid concentrate made of berries, cherries, or grapes, or perhaps a combination of all three. These superfoods are extremely high in antioxidant compounds called proanthocyanidins, which are known to facilitate wound healing.[15] They appear to do this, in part, by increasing the process of angiogenesis, the creation of new blood vessels that are needed for the initial phase of wound healing. They also limit inflammation and oxidative stress, along with the associated tissue damage, help improve local circulation, and help promote a strong collagen matrix, providing strength and resilience to newly formed tissues.[16] When a grape seed extract was applied to the skin wounds (surgical incisions) inflicted on the backs of mice, the wounds contracted and closed more rapidly.[17] And just as important, these natural agents are free of the potentially serious side effects that come with the long-term use of corticosteroids and nonsteroidal anti-inflammatory drugs like ibuprofen.

You can obtain grape seed extract as well as the berry, grape, or cherry concentrates from various sources on the Internet or through your local health food store. Be sure to dilute with water and also consider mixing whey protein powder into the beverage before you drink it. Of course, consuming the whole foods—fresh blueberries and cherries, for example—is an excellent way to obtain these

Table 7.2. Approximate Protein Content of Selected Foods

Foods	Protein Content/Serving Size
Fish (cod, sole, haddock, flounder)	21 grams/3 ounces
Salmon (sockeye)	23 grams/3 ounces
Shrimp	18 grams/3 ounces
Chicken	21 grams/3 ounces
Turkey, light meat	25 grams/3 ounces
Large egg	7 grams/egg
Cow's milk	8 grams/cup
Whey powder	20 grams/heaping tablespoon
Yogurt, low fat	12 grams/8 ounces
Yogurt, whole milk	8 grams/8 ounces
Cheese (e.g. Cheddar)	7 grams/ounce
Black-eyed peas (cooked)	12 grams/2 ounces
Kidney beans	11 grams/2 ounces
Lentils	6 grams/2 ounces
Tofu	8 grams/3.5 ounces
Peanuts	7 grams/ounce
Cashews	5 grams/ounce
Green beans (snap)	1.55 grams/cup
Broccoli (cooked)	4.5 grams/cup
Artichokes	6 grams/cup
Brussels sprouts (cooked)	5.5 grams/cup
Asparagus (cooked)	5 grams/cup
Bread	4 grams/slice
Wheat flour, whole grain	8 grams/half cup
Barley, pearled, raw	9 grams/half cup
Couscous	11 grams/half cup
Cornmeal	6 grams/half cup
Buckwheat flour	7.5 grams/half cup

antioxidant wonders as well. The concentrates just make it much easier to get this proanthocyanidin-rich support on a daily basis.

Nutritional assessment. Your physician or health provider may suggest a routine assessment of your nutritional status, though ideally this is also done *before* the operation. A standard assessment includes physical characteristics such as age, sex, height, and weight; a urine test for ketone bodies, urea, and creatinine; and blood tests for albumin, pre-albumin, iron, phosphate, and urea concentrations. More detailed assessments might include listing your usual dietary habits and measuring your blood levels of various nutrients. A registered dietitian can then help determine what steps to take to correct any deficiencies. Until you have such an assessment, you should continue to take the multiple as recommended in chapter 4.

Once you have made sure that your diet consists of wholesome nourishing foods, you should turn your attention to the supplements that will be helpful in the postoperative period. One of the ways you know your body is being stressed after surgery is a rise in body temperature, indicating inflammation. For every degree of temperature above normal, your nutritional needs increase by approximately 10 percent following minor surgery and by about 20 percent following major surgery.[18]

Moreover, as you will see, many of the nutrients, phytonutrients, and nutriceuticals mentioned in this chapter have specific effects on the healing process that cannot be provided by conventional medications.

❧ Using Supplements to Control Inflammation

In the previous chapter, we introduced you to the surgical stress response and some of its more troubling effects. A general part of this response is the inflammatory process. In the days following major surgery, there is a lot of inflammation around the surgical wound, as well as other areas of the body. This inflammation, as we noted earlier, in itself is not a bad thing, and, indeed, the wound healing process could not occur without it. A short-term, localized inflammatory response is helpful because it brings more nutrients and immune cells to the area, while also speeding up the removal of debris and toxins. But inflammation that spreads too far and lasts too long—that is, chronic, systemic inflammation—can be detrimental and will actually weaken the wound-healing process while also leaving you more vulnerable to pain and anxiety.

The first step toward reducing your body's tendency to become overly inflamed is to make certain dietary changes. Here, the type of fats you consume is crucial. After you've learned to avoid the proinflammatory fats (such as corn oil, safflower oil, sunflower oil, and partially hydrogenated "trans" fats), consider adding the anti-inflammatory supplements recommended below.

A variety of nutritional and herbal anti-inflammatory agents can help you keep chronic inflammation in check. We have summarized the main supplements of choice in Tables 7.3 and 7.4. The main herbal anti-inflammatories we recommend are curcumin, boswellia, bromelain, and holy basil. The main anti-inflammatory nutrients we recommend include an omega-3 supplement (either EPA or fish oil) and gamma-linolenic acid (GLA), which is actually an omega-6 fatty acid. Others may be included as well, of course, but these six agents are part of the core approach to the natural control of inflammation.

If you've just gone through major surgery, you should rely first on the anti-inflammatory medications your physician prescribes to "cool down" the initial surge of inflammatory chemicals in your body. Ice and elevation may also help during this postoperative period of intense inflammation. After a few days, switch over to the natural strategies introduced in this section, keeping in mind that these supplements tend to have more moderate anti-inflammatory effects unless used at high doses. Consult with a health care professional who understands the use of these natural agents before combining them on your own.

Many of the nutrients listed in Table 7.4 may be combined in the form of a "multiple." This is a much more practical way to obtain the benefits they provide. We recommend taking the multiple in combination with an herbal anti-inflammatory formula that has one or more of the herbs listed in Table 7.3. Many such formulas are now available in your local health food store. Whenever possible, check to see if the supplement has standardized ingredients and is produced by a reputable company.

Using supplements to create new healthy tissue. Within a week or two of surgery, the body's response to surgical stress has begun to cool down. Inflammation should be well under control by now. The mechanisms of tissue repair are in high gear, peaking at between 2 and 3 weeks after the surgery. Even while the inflammatory response is going on, the cells below the deepest skin layer, or dermis, begin to increase the production of new connective tissue. Connective tissue is simply the material in your body that supports other tissues and binds them together. This includes the bone, blood, and lymph tissues in addition to all the tissues that give support and structure to your skin and internal organs.

The central focus of new connective tissue formation is *collagen,* the body's most abundant protein. Cells called *fibroblasts* produce this protein at a rapid clip af-

Table 7.3. Herbal Supplements for Controlling Inflammation*

Supplement	Basic Anti-inflammatory Effect	Practical Notes
Curcumin (from the East Indian spice, turmeric)	In addition to anti-inflammatory effects, curcumin has antioxidant, digestive, antiplatelet, anticancer, and cholesterol-lowering effects.	400–600 mg three times a day; this is often combined with bromelain to enhance absorption; if taken as turmeric, take 4 tsp per day.
Boswellia	Complements the activity of curcumin and other anti-inflammatories, especially those known as COX-2 inhibitors; also excellent for bronchial asthma.	500 mg, 2 to 3 times per day, as the standardized root extract; for stronger inflammation, 3 grams, 3 times per day.
Bromelain and other proteolytic enzymes	This proteolytic enzyme helps remove fibrin, a clotting substance that prolongs inflammation; also breaks down other blood proteins that may cause chronic inflammation.	Bromelain: 500 mg three times per day, with food; often best combined with other proteolytic enzymes such as papain and pancreatin.
Holy basil (*Ocimum sanctum*, tulsi)	Contains phytonutrients that have a significant anti-inflammatory impact.	Take as directed on the label.
Other botanicals	Other anti-inflammatory herbs include ginger, garlic, hops, skullcap, feverfew, gotu kola, hawthorn, ginkgo, licorice, stinging nettle, bupleurum, goldenseal, green tea, lobelia, devil's claw, and calendula.	Consult with your physician or with an herbalist if you'd like to experiment with these other herbals; do not take these herbal supplements if you are already on anti-inflammatory or blood-thinning medication.

Supplement	Basic Anti-inflammatory Effect	Practical Notes
Berries, grapes, cherries (also available as liquid concentrate)	The anthocyanidins and proanthocyanidins in these fruits have strong anti-inflammatory effects and show a special affinity for connective tissue and collagen, promoting regeneration and tissue stability.	Consume these freely, as there is no known dosage limit; if taken as a liquid concentrate, be sure to dilute with water and consume on an empty stomach (15–20 minutes before solid food).

*Before using consult with your physician or with a health care professional who is well versed in herbal medicine and medicinal chemistry, especially if you are already taking anti-inflammatory drugs or blood-thinning medication.

Table 7.4. *Nutritional Agents for Controlling Inflammation*

Supplement	Basic Anti-inflammatory Effect	Practical Notes (dosage per day)
EPA	Eicosapentanoic acid, or EPA, an omega-3 fatty acid, can strongly decrease inflammation when used over a period of weeks.	2–3 g, with meals; take this for three months before switching to fish oil for three months, and then to fish oil plus borage oil (see below).
Fish oil	Fish oil contains both EPA and docosahexanoic acid (DHA), which has a more moderate impact on inflammation.	2–9 g, depending on body weight and degree of inflammatory imbalance; always consume with food.

continued

Supplement	Basic Anti-inflammatory Effect	Practical Notes (dosage per day)
Borage, evening primrose, black currant oil	These plant oils provide gamma-linolenic acid (GLA),which mildly decreases inflammation.	1–2 g; lower doses (1 gram or less) are recommended for long-term use; borage oil is an excellent complement to fish oil; primrose is better for women.
Vitamin C	This water-soluble vitamin has very mild anti-inflammatory effects; it can decrease histamine levels and therefore reduce allergic symptoms (allergies may perpetuate chronic inflammation).	2–6 g, in divided doses; doses higher than 5 g can lead to diarrhea, which can be avoided by gradually increasing the dosage (1 g on the first day, 2 g the second day, etc.) and taking divided doses over the course of the day.
Vitamin E	This micronutrient has very mild anti-inflammatory and anti-allergy effects.	400–600 IU per day, preferably as "mixed tocopherols" (different forms of vitamin E in combination); also may be included as part of a multiple.
Alpha-lipoic acid	This antioxidant works very well with vitamins C and E and other antioxidants to help combat inflammation.	300–1,200 mg; ideally, take in divided doses of 300 mg throughout the day.
N-acetyl cysteine (NAC)	This amino acid may help curb chronic inflammation when used in combination with the other agents listed here.	500–1,000 mg; do not exceed this amount, as higher doses may increase inflammation.

Supplement	Basic Anti-inflammatory Effect	Practical Notes (dosage per day)
Selenium	This trace element should be used in organic form (also called organoselenium), due to greater anti-inflammatory power than the inorganic forms.	150–250 mcg; selenium is synergistic with vitamin E, so the two are best taken in tandem.
Taurine	This semi-essential amino acid lowers the production of proinflammatory chemicals (cytokines).	1,500 mg in divided doses (500 mg, three times a day).

Note: If you are already taking anti-inflammatory drugs or blood-thinning medication, first consult with your physician or with a health care professional who is well versed in nutritional pharmacology. Since EPA and fish oil supplements are increasingly used for cardiovascular disease, surgeons must be wary of patients who are taking these supplements around the time of surgery.

ter surgery (or any form of tissue injury), providing it where strength, structure, and elasticity are needed. Collagen essentially functions as a kind of "scaffolding" for your body: it helps form a matrix or template for new tissue growth. It is essential to the structural integrity of any new tissue. The amount of collagen you produce during this time will determine the strength of your wound once it has healed.[19]

A number of nutrients can specifically influence the production of collagen in your body. The following supplements may be used as part of a multiple or as separate nutrient preparations to support your healing process right after surgery (once you've finished your medications or consulted with a physician to avoid unwanted reactions).

- **Vitamin C**. Vitamin C speeds up healing from fractures and other types of wounds.[20] It's also very important in counteracting the destructive effects of surgical stress, which explains why vitamin C is lost in the urine as a consequence of surgery.[21]

—Arnica and Post-Surgery Recovery—

Arnica montana is a perennial flower that has long been used for strains, sprains, swelling, and bruising. Arnica has mild anti-inflammatory, pain-relieving, and digestion-enhancing properties. It can be used topically in a 15 percent cream to decrease swelling and bruising, but it should not be used topically near cuts or surgical wounds. When taken orally, arnica must be used in homeopathic doses to avoid toxic effects. As a homeopathic remedy it is usually prescribed at the 30× dilution and used during the first two weeks after surgery.

A number of studies have been done with postsurgery patients taking arnica. Some studies have found a significant benefit in terms of a more rapid return to bowel function, decreased pain, and better overall recovery.[22] Nevertheless, the results have been rather mixed, with some studies showing no benefit, particularly in terms of alleviating bruising and hematoma after surgery. Though many people swear by arnica, more research is needed to determine its true usefulness. One of the practical dilemmas is that, in general, homeopathic arnica should not be taken concurrently with medications, as the therapeutic potential of the plant will be lost or greatly diminished. This fact may have affected the results of some studies.

Make sure you don't have an allergy to arnica before you take it; if you're allergic to sunflowers or marigolds, you may also be allergic to arnica. If you're interested in using arnica, consult with a licensed naturopathic or homeopathic physician in your area for a remedy that will be right for you.

With vitamin C, immediately following major surgery, a minimum dosage level of 2 to 3 g (2,000 to 3,000 mg) per day may be needed. A study out of the Department of Surgery at Carraway Methodist Medical Center in Birmingham, Alabama, found that patients who had undergone severe injuries or infection had deficient blood levels of vitamin C, averaging 0.11 mg/dl in the plasma throughout the day.[23] After two days of supplementing with 300 mg of vitamin C, the blood levels failed to increase. Over the next two days, the patients received 1,000 mg per day, and the blood levels began to improve. The researchers observed a significant increase in vitamin C levels following two days of supplementation at 3,000 mg (3 g) per day.

As a basic guideline, we suggest taking the two to three grams of vitamin C per day for the first three weeks after surgery. People who have undergone more serious injury or major surgery may even take as much as 4 g per day during the first week, then drop down to 3 g the second week, and 2 g the third week. After three months, 1 to 2 g per day may be sufficient to support postoperative healing and provide long-term maintenance.[24] Vitamin C is essential for the proper formation of collagen, proteoglycans, and other organic components of the connective tissues. Many studies indicate that the vitamin stimulates wound healing, strengthens your capillaries, and supports healthy immune function.[25] More serious surgical wounds may require large doses of vitamin C to support healing.[26] If you have a history of smoking and a stressful lifestyle, your vitamin C needs may be even higher.

- **Antioxidant multiple.** The antioxidant multiple we suggested for you in the preoperative period is even more important to use in the postsurgery period. If you do not keep oxidative stress under control, inflammation may become chronic and wound healing may not go smoothly.[27] This also may explain why antioxidant supplements have been proven to significantly reduce the risk of various post-op complications in heart surgeries as well as transplant surgeries.[28]

- **Vitamin A.** The vitamin A you started taking preoperatively is also important postoperatively. It is a cofactor in collagen formation and in the formation of a healthy, normal epithelium—the tissue that covers all the internal and external surfaces of the body.[29] Vitamin A may be provided as part of a multivitamin (15,000 to 25,000 IU/day) that also contains the B vitamins. Vitamin A can also be applied topically to avoid high levels of A in the bloodstream—something you'd want to do if you are planning a pregnancy or already pregnant, breast-feeding, or using steroid medications.

- **B complex.** The vitamins B_1, B_2, B_5, B_6, B_{12}, and folic acid all collaborate in the processes of cellular growth and metabolism. Vitamins B_1 and B_5 are also crucial for collagen synthesis, and vitamin B_5 can help increase your resilience to stress. Supplementing with folic acid, as well as vitamins B_6 and B_{12}, may help lower homocysteine levels, which tend to rise following some surgical situations.[30] (Homocysteine is an amino acid derived from protein-rich foods; high levels in the blood are a risk factor for coronary artery disease, dementia, and depression.) In people over age fifty, vitamin B_{12} injections have been known to help eliminate fatigue, weakness, mood swings, and appetite loss following surgery. Many of our patients have benefited by taking these before and after surgery in the practical form of a B-complex multivitamin (for dosage, take as directed on the label). Try not to take formulas containing vitamin B_6 in the evening, however, as some people find that it has a stimulatory effect and keeps them up at night.

- **Minerals and trace elements.** Zinc, copper, iron, and magnesium participate in thousands of enzyme reactions throughout the body at every moment of the day. These elements are needed to produce collagen and repair tissue.[31] There is excellent evidence that zinc does promote healing from surgery.[32] And since surgery itself seems to increase the body's requirements for zinc, it's important to get enough. A controlled clinical trial in France found that supplementing with zinc postsurgery, at a modest dose of 30 mg per day for three days, corrected the substantial drop in blood zinc levels that occurred immediately after the operation.[33] It also appeared that the blood levels of the stress hormone, cortisol, was among the factors that depleted the zinc supply. One might therefore predict that the stronger the stress response to surgery, the higher the body's needs for zinc after the operation.

    Additional zinc is needed for increased DNA and protein synthesis and to help stabilize cell membranes during tissue repair. Again, a good multivitamin-mineral supplement is the best way to go. Try to find one that provides between 15 and 30 mg of zinc per day. Higher doses (50 mg per day) may be recommended for people suffering from immune suppression, malnutrition, malabsorption, or chronic diarrhea. Do not exceed these doses, as excessive zinc tends to *impede* the healing process.[34] The same point can be made about copper, which is antagonistic to zinc.

- **Glutamine and arginine.** The amino acids glutamine and arginine (as well as others like methionine, histidine, serine, lysine, and asparagine) play key roles in wound healing and immune function.[35] Glutamine is recommended for people who have had surgeries that affect the digestive tract in particular, or those who have received either anti-inflammatory drugs or chemotherapy in the past. Arginine has been shown to increase collagen formation, blood flow to the wound area, and tissue repair.[36] We recommend supplementing with L-glutamine (5 to 30 g per day) and L-arginine (10 to 20 g per day) in the first two months following surgery. The higher doses can be helpful if you're suffering from infection, suppressed immunity, and considerable weight loss following surgery.[37] Caution: Do not take arginine if you have cancer, as it may stimulate the growth of some tumors. This and other amino acids, such as L-lysine, should be used as a supplement for no more than 6 months. Glutamine can be added to the Power Healing Drink. A scoop of flax fiber powder— for example, FiberSMART by ReNew Life—contains a combination of ingredients that support bowel function (glutamine, lactobacillus, etc.) and can be added to the Power Healing Drink daily.

- **Gotu kola (*Centella asiatica*, madecassol).** Gotu kola has been used as a therapeutic herb in many parts of the world. Traditional herbalists in China and India have long praised the herb for enhancing the healing of wounds. Gotu kola and its components have been shown to stimulate collagen production, improve wound healing, and reduce excessive scarring following surgery.[38] Anecdotal claims have been made for better sleep, improved memory, and more sustained energy levels. A normal daily dose is about 600 mg of the dried leaves or infusion. The single-dose capsules are typically 400 mg and can be taken two to three times daily. Alternatively, a 10 mg concentrated extract, also available in capsules, may be taken three times daily. Look for an extract standardized to contain 30 to 40 percent of the triterpene compounds, including asiaticoside, asiatic acid, madecassic acid, and madecassoside.

- **Bromelain.** Bromelain refers to a family of proteolytic enzymes derived from pineapple. Numerous studies have found that taking bromelain supplements has led to the reduction of edema, bruising, pain, and healing time following surgery.[39] Aside from its well-documented anti-inflammatory activity, bromelain supplementation may also lead to more rapid disappearance of hematoma (blood pooling under the skin), pain, and swelling after surgery.[40] The recommended adult dose is 500 mg two to four times each day beginning a few days before surgery.[41] Nonetheless, because of bromelain's blood-thinning properties, it may be safer to start using the supplement immediately *after* surgery, not before. (Again, wait until the postmedication period before you start this.) As long as you're not allergic to pineapple, there should be no side effects, even with very high doses.

- **Aloe vera.** We tend to take the healing effects of aloe vera for granted. Many of us, at one time or another have broken off a stalk of aloe vera plant and dabbed it on a wound. Nonetheless, scientific studies have only recently begun to confirm the usefulness of this plant. Both internal and external use of aloe vera may be helpful in speeding up tissue repair and improving immune function after surgery.[42] There is some rather striking preliminary evidence that aloe vera can speed up wound healing in diabetics, a population that typically is slow to heal after surgery.[43] The recommended doses depend on the concentration and therefore vary greatly—from 1 to 2 tablespoons to a full cup of aloe juice or more. Aloe preparations that are bottled close to the source of harvest are most concentrated in the primary active ingredient, called acemannan. Few aloe products on the market are processed in this way. Try to find aloe products that have had the anthraquinones removed; these are laxative substances that can lead to diarrhea following surgery.

Topical application of both aloe vera and gotu kola extracts to surgical scars or wounds may also facilitate the repair process. Aloe vera gel is widely used for this purpose, and it has been shown to dramatically increase the collagen content of wounds.[44] Although more clinical trials are needed to determine the safety and benefits of these two supplements at high doses, they are clearly safe enough to be applied topically, and their oral use is supported by centuries of therapeutic claims by practitioners of traditional Asian medicine. At least some of their reported benefits may also be due to their anti-inflammatory and antioxidant properties.[45]

As you can see, different nutritional and herbal supplements can have a positive influence on tissue repair as well as limit the damaging effects of inflammation. During the tissue repair process, we also recommend avoiding high doses of omega-6 fatty acids from corn oil, safflower oil, and animal products, as well as high doses of fish oil and vitamins D and E. There is some laboratory evidence that these nutrients can interfere with normal tissue healing when taken in high doses. One possible explanation is that high doses of these nutrients may block the formation of new blood vessels (angiogenesis), which is essential for wound healing. Clinical studies are needed to test this hypothesis.

We'll talk more about vitamin E here, since so many people already take the vitamin. The use of vitamin E cream largely has been ineffective as a way to speed up the healing of skin or to improve its appearance. One well-designed clinical trial found no benefit to the cosmetic outcome of scars by applying vitamin E cream after skin surgery; and in some cases, the vitamin E seemed to worsen the cosmetic appearance of a scar.[46] Therefore, we recommend against the use of topical vitamin E after surgery. Topical applications of aloe vera, gotu kola, comfrey, or calendula (an excellent ointment for controlling inflammation and promoting tissue repair) are a much better choice.

Supplemental vitamin E hasn't been shown to have a consistent beneficial effect on tissue repair. The results of studies with laboratory animals receiving vitamin E either orally or by injection have been mixed, with some research actually showing inhibition of wound healing, some showing no effect, and others showing improved wound healing.[47] Of particular concern is research that says vitamin E may block or retard the repair of tendons.[48] Because of the inconsistent results, we do not recommend taking a vitamin E supplement separately after surgery. If you're taking an antioxidant multiple, the amount of vitamin E contained in it is not likely to have any negative effect, and it may even help reinforce the effects of other nutrients.

✇ Sleeping to Heal and Reenergize

People often complain after surgery that they feel exhausted. This is simply the body's way of asking for sleep, the body's way of requesting the space and time it needs to let the repair process move forward unhindered. Rest or sleep enables the body to concentrate its energies on healing the wound and restoring function.

The main biochemical benefit of sleep is a surge of growth hormone.[49] (It is a kind of yin-yang irony that exercise is the other major stimulus for growth hormone production.) This hormone may be called the master healing hormone: it helps drive protein synthesis and thus the formation of new tissue. About 70 percent of the total 24-hour secretion of growth hormone occurs during sleep.[50] Most of the growth hormone is being released during the first two hours, the period known as "deep sleep." This appears to be the most critical period for healing.

The younger you are, the more growth hormone you produce during sleep. As you get older—and especially after age forty-five—your production of growth hormone drops off, as does the amount of deep sleep you experience at night.[51] Anything that interferes with that sleep will tend to dampen the growth hormone response, and weaken the body's self-healing potential in the process.[52]

This helps us understand why the tissue repair process becomes less efficient as we grow older. It also helps drive home the fact that, in order to heal efficiently, you need to get plenty of sleep and take a vacation from the demands and pressures of daily life. Too often people are juggling so many responsibilities at work and home that they end up with a health problem requiring surgery. And yet as soon as they open their eyes after the surgery, they expect to begin the juggling act all over again. So, too, does everyone else they know.

This is a dangerous pattern, and it will not be conducive to a smooth recovery. To heal you must give yourself permission to slow down and chill out for a few days. Too much busy activity following the operation will divert your healing energies from the task at hand. So take a break from your busy routines in order to heal. Let someone else be the organizer. Hang up the "do not disturb" sign, and give yourself plenty of time before trying to return to being as active as you were before surgery.

Unfortunately, certain medications can also interfere with sleep, and these can work against you when you're trying to deepen your sleep with some of the natural strategies. Many of our patients have found that a combination of gentle herbal sedatives—valerian, hops, passionflower, and lemon balm—helped lessen the sleep-disrupting effects of some medications. These and other natural sleep aides, such as the amino acid 5-hydroxytryptophan (5-HTP), are now widely available in health food stores.[53] The 5-HTP, which we mentioned in chapter 6, can be especially beneficial for people under age fifty. Try different combinations of supplements and see what works for you.

For people over age fifty, a melatonin tablet (1 to 3 mg per night) can be a very helpful way to deepen your sleep and enhance your body's self-healing potential. In addition to enhancing sleep quality, melatonin stimulates many aspects of the immune response, inhibits tumor invasion, and protects against viral infections.[54] Melatonin levels can often be altered by the altered sleep patterns that occur with hospitalization (awakenings for vital sign checks and medications). You can have your melatonin levels checked to see if you're producing enough at night. Chances are that if you're sleeping poorly, your melatonin rhythms are going to be askew as well. Taking a time-release melatonin supplement at a regular time each night, ideally between 10 and 11 p.m., or one-half hour before you turn in, can work wonders under these circumstances.

Last, don't forget to adopt good sleep habits: avoiding or greatly minimizing your caffeine intake during the day, avoiding alcohol and big meals in the evening, avoiding computer screens and bright lights at night, sleeping in pitch dark, getting to bed well before midnight, getting out in sunlight or full-spectrum light in the morning, exercising during the day, and practicing relaxation techniques to prevent the high-pressure arena of daily life from creeping into your nighttime reverie. All of these habits will help improve your sleep quality, and any one of them can make a significant difference.

❧ Be Gentle with Your Body

Remember that it can take several weeks to recover from the physical challenges posed by major surgery. Although most incisions close within a few days and heal within a week, at least to the point where you can begin moving around, heed your physician's advice regarding physical activity. In most cases, walking and gentle cycling are allowed within a short period of time. Nonetheless, be sure to get your doctor's permission before engaging in light exercise or lifting anything that weighs over 10 pounds. Any heavy lifting or other kinds of strenuous activity should be avoided within the first few weeks after major surgery.

—Exercise Tips after Surgery—

While "taking it slow" and resting are good ideas after major surgery, so, too, is exercise in moderation. The trick is to find a level of intensity that is not too stressful. During your recovery phase, it's best to exercise at a fat-burning heart rate (beats per minute should approximately equal 170 minus your chronological age) rather than the much faster cardiorespiratory training rate. The more moderate level of exercise intensity will be less likely to trigger the sympathetic nervous system and the stress response. If in doubt, find an exercise trainer or exercise physiologist to work with so that you understand the ideal target heart rate and how to monitor it.

Be sure to give your body time to build up to a level of exertion, and then give it time to recover after a vigorous workout before you exercise again. Your physician, physical therapist, or exercise physiologist can advise you on the kinds of activity that won't cause your body too much stress in the weeks following the operation.

While it's not necessary to partake in formal exercise regimens, we do encourage you to find something that resembles a gentle workout. You might begin by joining your local YMCA, fitness center, or country club simply to have access to the swimming pool. Regular swimming is the perfect activity for many people in postsurgery recovery, because it's so gentle on the

---

joints yet works the muscles and cardiovascular system. Swimming with increasing effort to *gradually* increase your heart rate and stimulate your muscle activity is readily accomplished. Water aerobics is for many people a better activity than land-based aerobics classes because aquatic activities are so much easier on the body. But don't forget to think simple by integrating activity into your daily life. Examples of everyday activities that can help you get back up to speed with your overall fitness include:

- Brisk walking, but only at your own pace
- Taking the stairs, not the elevator
- Gardening, because digging and weeding are good for you!
- Golfing without a cart—even if your golfing buddies don't follow suit
- Dancing to any music that moves you
- Tennis, either singles or doubles, though the latter tends to be easier on the body
- Jogging, alternating with walking
- Mowing and cleaning up the lawn
- Riding a bike, whether stationary or mobile
- Playing Frisbee, tag, and other outdoor kid games
- Housecleaning and other home maintenance endeavors

❧ Safe and Effective Support for Growth Hormone Production

Far from giving out under the strain of wear and tear, the human body is designed to hold up astonishingly well. It is naturally endowed with remarkable powers of renewal, self-repair, and regeneration. The secret to unlocking these powers lies not in genetic tinkering or a high-tech fix, but in supporting Mother Nature at what she does best: restoring order after chaos. Surgery triggers a process of extreme breakdown, something known as *hypercatabolism*. It's like a form of accelerated aging: energy levels decline, immune function falters, and muscles atrophy. Under these conditions, it also becomes more difficult to *rebuild* muscle, which only increases a feeling of weakness and fatigue over time.

The way to stop and reverse this process is to encourage the body's ability to repair and rebuild itself—the marvelous process known as *anabolism*. Although medicine does provide certain anabolic agents—such as growth hormone (GH), insulin-like growth factor, DHEA, and synthetic forms of testosterone—to support this essential restorative force, such agents can have serious risks and side effects. They are best used only for a short amount of time, in conjunction with nutrition and exercise.[55]

What's more, many of the anabolic benefits of GH can be obtained through lifestyle adjustments alone and through targeted use of specific amino acids, the building blocks of protein. What follows are some examples of how you can optimize your *anabolic power,* the body's ability to repair and rebuild itself.

- *Maintain optimum nutrition*. Without good nutrition, GH levels are likely to decline more rapidly with age, a process that starts at age twenty-one.[56] Simply consuming an adequate amount of protein and calories is one of the prerequisites for a healthy anabolic response.[57] But eating too much fat, especially saturated fats and hydrogenated fats, will tend to decrease your GH levels. Antioxidants in the diet—from vegetables, berries, cherries, and grapes—will help to keep the pituitary gland in good working order for robust GH production.

- *Reduce your consumption of refined carbohydrates*. White sugar, brown sugar, corn syrup, high-fructose corn syrup, and white flour products all raise insulin levels, and elevated blood insulin levels may tend to lower GH secretion by the pituitary.[58] The effect is strongest when you consume refined carbohydrates on an empty stomach. Whenever feasible, hold off on that hospital Jell-O until you've had a chance to put something more wholesome in your belly.

- *Consider using a "GH releaser" supplement*. Diet alone cannot provide the support you need for maximum anabolic power. Supplementing with specific combinations of amino acids, taken at night on an empty stomach, can help coax the pituitary gland to secrete more youthful levels of GH.[59] These so-called GH releasers (substances that trigger the secretion of growth hormone) can boost protein synthesis, improve body composition, and further enhance tissue repair—in some cases quite dramatically. All of the GH releaser supplements now on the market include the amino acids arginine, lysine, ornithine, and glutamine, along with the branched-chain amino acids, leucine, isoleucine, and valine. What make these products different from one another are the specific ratios of amino acids, the quality of the protein source, and whether there are any additional ingredients such as herbal agents. We prefer ones with no additional ingredients and organically grown plants (e.g., soybean) as the protein source.*

- *Intensify your workout routine.* Once your surgeon has given you the ok to return to more vigorous exercise, you might try taking your workout to a higher level of intensity. Increasing the duration or intensity of your exercise routine can result in a potent boost in GH production.[60] This has been demonstrated in people of all ages, but the benefits may be greatest for older or elderly people who tend to have lower GH levels compared to younger people.[61] Again, if you're just getting in shape after a long period of inactivity, you may want to work with a physical therapist, personal trainer, or exercise physiologist to help you work up to the proper level of exertion.

- *Limit your alcohol intake.* Drinking alcohol on a regular basis disrupts the GH anabolic signal, apparently by directly affecting the liver.[62] Most surgeries will require you to stay away from alcohol for one to two weeks after the surgery. Even after this point, however, it's best for the healing process to drink in moderation. Try to avoid drinking any alcoholic beverage (even beer or wine) on an empty stomach.

---

* When selecting an HGH releaser, purchase only those that contain pure amino acids derived from plant sources. There should be no added ingredients, herbal or otherwise. Many HGH releasers on the market contain various stimulants; in addition, the amino acids are derived from bacterial synthesis rather than plant sources. Only plant-derived amino acids seem to provide long-lasting effectiveness. In the appendix, we list reputable sources for these and other supplements.

- *Get a good night's sleep.* As we discussed earlier on page 190, sleep and healing are inseparable. Good sleep is essential to GH production and thus to your body's ability to repair damaged tissue and build new tissues.[63]

Simply by getting enough exercise and sleep, you can begin to increase your body's ability to repair and rebuild itself. With diet and nutritional supplementation, you can further enhance your anabolic power, shifting your metabolism in a healthier direction. By following the guidelines laid out in this handbook, you should be able to do just that. Whereas surgery tends to make your metabolism sluggish, a hallmark sign of premature aging, our guidelines will help you shift your body toward a more vital, rejuvenating metabolism.

In this chapter, we have introduced you to a program that can support rapid repair. Some of these recommendations will likely exert a stronger influence on your self-healing ability than others. For this reason, we recommend that you explore at least three of the supplement options we have laid out for preventing inflammation and enhancing the formation of new tissue. Remember that eating a good diet, getting plenty of rest and exercise, and managing your stress are also just as important, if not more so. You must see your life as a whole, avoiding those factors that interfere with wound healing (high-fat diet, smoking, sugar, alcohol, etc.) while emphasizing all those factors that are conducive to tissue regeneration and repair.

If you decide to take the minimalist approach and use only a few of the supplements mentioned in this chapter, there is still a good chance you will benefit, depending on your particular situation—and, of course, whether you're sticking to a good diet as well. Nonetheless, if you've recently undergone major surgery and feel that you need additional support, larger combinations of supplements and higher dosages may be needed to have a positive impact on your recovery. If you're unsure about dosages or combinations, consult with a knowledgeable health care professional to get more clarity.

8

Holistic Support for Specific Surgical Scenarios

Full of sweet dreams, and health and quiet breathing.

—Keats

Jane M., a forty-five-year-old veterinarian and mother of three, came to my office with a large and painful ovarian cyst and a history of irritable bowel syndrome. Surgery was necessary to rule out cancer. And yet thanks to her training as a vet, she knew all too well the harmful effects anesthesia could have on digestion. She also conceded to a fear of surgery in general. "They wheel you away from your loved ones, from all your possessions," she told me. "You can't even wear your own clothes or glasses. It just seems like death to me."

We then discussed what could be done to make the surgery a more life-affirming event to her. I offered to walk with Jane as she left her family in the pre-op waiting room. I suggested that she keep her glasses on until she went to sleep, and then agreed to keep them in my pocket, returning them to her after the surgery, as soon as she emerged from the anesthesia. I also instructed the recovery room staff to have Jane's family by her bedside as soon as she awoke and appeared stable. Fear of not being able to see them when she came to seemed to lie at the heart of Jane's anxieties. With a smile, but also a hint of trepidation in her eyes, she told me she agreed with the plan.

Next, we began exploring options for getting Jane fit for surgery. She and I worked together to bolster her nutritional approach, following the core recommendations laid down in chapter 4. Because her need for surgery was urgent, she only had 10 days to implement the Rapid Recovery Program. Still, she immediately took to the Power Healing Drink and was already using a good multivitamin and omega-3 supplements. She had also received acupuncture several times and practiced progressive muscle relaxation almost daily, and she planned to continue with these practices right up to the surgery, in order to minimize nausea, constipation, and intestinal pain. Having her glasses on before the anesthesia took hold, while she was still awake, seemed to help her feel more in control and less stressed.

For the elective surgery, I used a laparoscopic approach that minimized stress to Jane's intestines. She wore acupressure wristbands and received preventive nausea medication from her anesthesiologist. In the operating room, I eased her into a more relaxed state with a deep breathing exercise along with several hypnotic suggestions (described in chapter 5) to help her relax further and to restore good bowel function.

To our collective relief, the ovary turned out to be free of cancer. Instead, Jane had an endometriosis cyst, which I was able to remove with relative ease.

That afternoon, Jane returned home with her loving family, and later that evening she ate a full meal, with no digestive upset whatsoever. She continued with the Power Healing Drink and took lactobacillus and glutamine supplements to further promote her intestinal health. It is typical for patients with irritable bowel syndrome to have significant flare-ups in their symptoms following abdominal or pelvic surgery. But Jane felt great and experienced no disruption of her digestion. Within two weeks, she had completely recovered and was back to her work as an animal doctor.

—EGM

As you can see from Jane's example, there are a number of ways to fine-tune your approach to a specific surgical situation. Every scenario involves special considerations in terms of diet, supplements, and other aspects of care. In this chapter, we will explore a few of the more common scenarios, with an emphasis on the region of the body that is most affected and how to protect and repair that part of the body. For example, prostate, uterine, and intestinal surgeries all pertain to the abdomen/pelvic area, while joint reconstruction and hip replacement pertain to the musculoskeletal system.

Accordingly, we focus on a core set of integrative strategies for each of the following five major areas: abdomen/pelvic area, cardiothoracic system, musculoskeletal system, nervous system, and immune system. Keep in mind that the advice we provide here is intended only as a kind of checklist for you to explore with your physician and caregivers. A full rationale for each checklist is beyond the scope of this chapter. Nonetheless, we will try to give you a flavor of some of the thinking that goes into the decision-making process for following these suggestions.

In this chapter, we introduce you to additional supplements that can be used for specific types of surgery, either to promote healing or reduce the risk of post-operative complications, or both. Try to use the checklists as a complement to the core supplement program outlined in chapters 4 (pre-op) and 7 (post-op). By taking these supplements before and after your operation, you will support the healing process and diminish post-operative pain and discomfort.

For most of the supplements listed below, we provide dosage ranges within which you can find the right dose for you. The FDA does not regulate most of these agents as drugs; therefore the proper doses may vary considerably from one brand to the next, and quality and quantity of active ingredients may vary as well. Many come in different forms, including tablets, tinctures, and teas. Instead of guessing your particular dosage needs, it can be helpful to consult with a health care professional well versed in the use of nutrients and nutriceuticals when deciding on a particular dosage and manufacturer. Appropriate and safe doses for pregnant and breast-feeding women may not be known for many of these agents, though some guidelines do exist. For example, pregnant women should avoid goldenseal and many other herbs; also, their daily intake of vitamin A should not exceed 2,500 IU per day, while 4,000 IU is okay for nursing mothers.

In some cases, you may want to undergo biochemical testing to help figure out whether a particular supplement or combination of nutrients should be taken at higher doses. For example, if your blood level of homocysteine is elevated following surgery, the temporary use of high-dose folic acid (3 to 5 mg per day) and vitamin B6 (200 to 400 mg per day) may be helpful. High levels of methylmalonic acid in your urine indicate the need for vitamin B_{12} supplementation. Simply measuring blood levels of various nutrients can also tell you whether you might want to supplement with these nutrients, though blood measures alone are usually inadequate because water-soluble vitamins like vitamin C are quickly excreted, and because of the body's complex strategies for regulating the levels of various nutrients.

Additionally, if you are taking any medications, please be aware of the potential for drug-nutrient interactions that can undermine the effectiveness of your medications. The reverse relationship is also possible: certain drugs may alter the metabolism of certain nutrients. For example, tetracycline and thyroid medications tend to increase excretion of calcium, while heparin interferes with the activation of vitamin D, resulting in osteopenia (chronic bone loss). There are now databases available that can tell you about these interactions and whether it is safe to supplement when you're also taking medication. One example is the IBIS (Interactive Body-Mind Information System) database, which can be found at www.ibismedical.com.

In terms of drug-supplement interactions that occur during surgery, the two most serious concerns are increased bleeding and intensified effects of anesthesia, causing the body to be overly sedated after surgery (see Table 8.1).[1] Also, if taken while under anesthesia, herbs can cause negative hormonal changes, clotting disorders, cardiovascular complications, water and electrolyte disturbances, and liver damage (hepatotoxicity).[2] Complicating this situation is the fact that a number of the drugs used for anesthesia also have blood-thinning effects. A recent case report suggested that sevoflurane (used in the administration of general anesthesia) when combined with aloe vera created an increased risk of excessive bleeding.[3]

Given these types of concerns, the American Society of Anesthesiologists has recommended that all herbal medications should be discontinued two to three weeks before an elective surgery.[4] One of the reasons for this strong precaution-

Table 8.1. Herbal Remedies: Potential Areas of Concern for Surgical Patients*

Herbs That May Inhibit Platelet Aggregation	Herbs That May Inhibit Clotting	Herbs That May Increase the Depressant Effects of Anesthesia	Miscellaneous Herbs of Potential Concern
Concern: Risk of hemorrhage when taken with NSAIDs or other blood-thinning drugs	*Concern: Potential for excessive bleeding during surgery*	*Concern: Potential prolonging of the sedative effects of anesthesia*	*Concerns: see comments below on echinacea, ephedra, and Saint-John's-wort*
Aloe vera	Chamomile	Hops	Echinacea affects immunosuppressive drugs, may cause liver damage when combined with antirheumatic drugs
Bilberry	Dandelion root	Kava kava	
Bromelain	Dong quai	Passionflower	
Devil's claw	Ginseng	Valerian	
Dong quai	Horse chestnut		
Feverfew			
Fish oil			Ephedra can cause cardiac stress, stroke
Flaxseed oil			
Garlic			
Ginger			Saint-John's-wort alters the metabolism of many drugs
Ginkgo			
Grapeseed extract			

* These lists may not be comprehensive; databases are being constantly updated to accommodate new scientific findings on these agents. Issues related to tolerance and withdrawal effects are still to be determined for most of these agents in the context of anesthesia.

ary stance is that very few anesthesiologists have a detailed knowledge and understanding of the potential risks of herbal medicines. We recommend that you consult with a physician well-versed in herbal therapies and integrative medicine before using any of these herbs before surgery. Most will be safe to restart once anesthesia has worn off, all epidurals have been removed, bleeding is well controlled, and you have returned to a regular diet (24 to 72 hours).

❧ Surgeries Involving the Abdomen/Pelvic Area

> *Roger, an aspiring architect in his early twenties, had undergone an emergency appendectomy in August. After recovering fairly well from his surgery, over the holidays he had lifted some heavy boxes and suddenly began to feel pain in the abdomen where the incision had been made. Roger really wanted to avoid narcotic pain medications because they made him feel nauseous. When I examined him during his first visit to our office in January, I found tenderness in several key points (called trigger points) around two out of three surgical scars. I confirmed that he did not have a hernia.*
>
> *Initially, Roger's pain was rated 7 on a scale of 1 to 10. I offered him osteopathic manipulation of his abdomen and local anesthetic injection of the trigger points. After the osteopathic treatment and injections, the intensity of his pain had dropped down to 2. I then taught him some stretches and reviewed strategies for lifting. He did very well after this and never needed any medication stronger then Advil. I did not see him in the office again until the next January when he returned from a ski vacation.*
>
> *—TMM*

Classic examples of abdominal/pelvis surgery include appendectomy, oophorectomy, hysterectomy, gastric bypass surgery, and prostatectomy. The main physical functions often affected by these surgeries are digestive, sexual, and bladder/kidney function. In addition, the liver and pancreas, both part of the gastrointestinal system, can become markedly stressed by major surgery. In this regard, a recent study found that fish oil supplementation after major abdominal surgery resulted in better functioning of the liver and pancreas; this protection resulted in a more rapid recovery.[5] But again, most of the research suggests that you should begin supplementation with omega-3 fats (fish oil or EPA) and glutamine for at least a month *before* the surgery.[6] (See "How Omega-3 Supplementation Helps You Prepare for Surgery," in chapter 4. Remember to stop taking the omega-3s one week before surgery to cut down on the risk of excessive bleeding.)

Acupuncturists often say that cutting into the abdomen or across the torso can have a detrimental impact on your vitality for many months after the operation. We have found that acupuncture, qigong, or other forms of so-called energy medicine can be very helpful in restoring health after major abdominal surgery. Therapeutic exercise can include restorative yoga and tai chi to help strengthen the abdominal area without strain.

As far as your digestion goes, here are supplements you can take to restore normal function.

- Glutamine, 10 to 20 g per day for first two to three weeks, then 3 to 5 g per day for two additional weeks (ideally combined with exercise)
- Aloe vera, 4 tbs or ½ cup per day; can have a cleansing effect on the colon when combined with psyllium husks
- L-acidophilus and other probiotics, particularly important if antibiotics or chemotherapy was used in the recent past
- Omega-3 fatty acids (fish oil): 4 to 8 g per day. Remember to begin supplementation at least a few weeks before surgery, but stop taking the omega-3s one week prior to the operation to avoid an increased risk of hemorrhage.
- Milk thistle (active component: silymarin): use as tincture, three dropperfuls in a glass of water, 2 to 3 times a day in the first week after surgery
- Digestive enzymes (betaine, papain, pacreatin, etc.)

Other natural remedies for digestive problems:

- Soluble and insoluble fiber, in water
- Qigong breathing (deep abdominal breathing and energy cultivation exercises from traditional Chinese medicine)
- Relaxation tapes to increase the parasympathetic response
- Hypnotic suggestions to minimize nausea and promote digestion
- Smaller meals, well-cooked high-fiber meals, vegetable soups

Natural strategies for restoring sexual vitality and potency include (dosages for supplements are daily unless we indicate otherwise):

- Vitamin B_6: 50 to 100 mg
- Magnesium: 400 mg twice
- Zinc: 15 mg for women, 30 mg for men
- Asian ginseng and other tonifying herbs
- Acupuncture
- Vigorous but not overly strenuous exercise (including sex)
- Cultivate peace and harmony with your partner

Natural strategies for restoring female fertility include:

- Vitamin B_6: 50 to 100 mg
- Multi-mineral/vitamin supplement (high in antioxidant nutrients)
- Adrenal insufficiency: consider adrenal supplements along with vitamin C and pantothenic acid
- Acupuncture
- Acetyl-L-carnitine: 1 g three times a day
- Arginine: 2 g twice a day
- Zinc picolinate: 30 to 60 mg
- Magnesium: 400 mg twice a day
- EPA (omega-3): 1 to 3 g
- Vitamin E: 400 I.U. twice a day
- Vitamin C: 1 g three times a day
- L-arginine: 4 g
- Coenzyme Q10: 60 mg

Natural strategies for restoring bladder/kidney function include:

- Cordyceps (medicinal mushrooms, take as directed)
- Berry, grape, and cherry concentrates
- Asian ginseng and other tonifying herbs
- Acupuncture
- Massage-based pain management for sacral nerves

Additional points for people undergoing abdominal surgery:

- **Shaving the wound area.** Many surgeries require that the hair on the skin where the incision is to be made be removed before the procedure. Clipping your hair, the night before surgery, helps avert the need for shaving. Clipping has a lower risk or skin infection then shaving does. If you cannot clip, then shaving the area on the day of the surgery, rather than the night before, will lower the risk of infection.

- **Choice of anesthesia: general versus regional.** It's helpful to review with your surgeon or anesthesiologist the different options for anesthesia. Many doctors prescribe general anesthesia because it's easier to administer and some patients do not like to be awake and immobile for the length of the surgery. Yet even with regional anesthesia, your anesthesiologist can control the amount of anesthesia so that you may doze off. But regional anesthesia (epidural block or spinal block) may result in a quicker recovery than general anesthesia, causes less stress on the heart and on the immune system, and avoids the paralyzing effects on the intestinal function associated with general anesthesia. It's also a good choice during pregnancy and breast-feeding because the developing child is exposed to far less medication. Regional anesthesia is not usually possible for most laparoscopic procedures but can be used in open abdominal pelvic surgeries.

- **Massage and manipulation before and after surgery.** Many hospitals now provide massage with therapeutic essential oils to promote relaxation before the surgery. If your hospital does not provide this service, consider scheduling a session with a licensed massage therapist who uses aromatherapy. After surgery, osteopathic manipulation has been shown to decrease complications such as blood clots and ileus (slow bowel function). Therapeutic touch and other gentle bodywork techniques can be performed in the hospital on the days following your procedure. Ask your doctor if this is available at your hospital.

- **Reproductive planning.** If your surgery involves the reproductive organs or genital area, it is very important to discuss with your doctor your reproductive plans, preferences for management of hormone withdrawal symptoms, and timing for safely returning to sexual activity.

- **Surgery, ovulation, and pregnancy.** Major surgery may disrupt normal ovulation for several cycles. Periods may become irregular especially if ovarian or uterine surgery is done. If this persists for more then two cycles, notify your physician. Practicing contraception prior to major surgery may be helpful to avoid anesthetic risks to a developing fetus and the strain on the mother of healing while carrying a pregnancy. Some surgeries cannot be avoided during pregnancy. Notify your physician and anesthesiologist if there is any chance you may be pregnant.

- **Tips on pelvic surgeries.** For many pelvic surgeries, your doctor may recommend pelvic rest for days to weeks after surgery. For women, this will mean nothing in the vagina, including tampons, douches, or intercourse. For men, this means avoiding intercourse. These guidelines are given to prevent infection or prevent straining stitches. Once these risks have past, sexual activity can resume. Gently using these muscles is important to restoring blood flow and promoting healing. Slight tension or tenderness may occur initially, and can be overcome with massage, position change, and gentleness. Pain should be reported to the physician and care should be taken not to traumatize the area.

✆ Surgeries Involving the Chest (Cardiothoracic)

Any surgery that involves your heart and circulatory system will qualify for this category. Classic examples of surgeries that affect this area include angioplasty, valve replacement, heart transplant, coronary bypass surgery, and any form of open-heart surgery. Surgery for sleep apnea (e.g., rhinoplasty) and removal of any cancer in the chest area (breast and lung tumors, for example) also can apply to this category. One could, in principle, lump the cardiovascular and pulmonary systems together because so many operations involving the chest area tend to impact both systems.

If you have a history of a heart murmur, you should notify your doctor, as you may need special antibiotics during surgery to protect the heart. Also be sure to notify your doctor if you are taking any blood-thinning medication, herbs, or supplements. Most of the aspirin- and ibuprofen-type medications should be stopped 7 days prior to elective surgery. For prescription medications, your surgeon will notify you if your medication should be stopped or substituted.

Natural strategies for improving or maintaining cardiovascular and cardiac function include (dosages for supplements are daily unless we indicate otherwise):

- Low-fat diet, avoidance of saturated fat and omega-6 fats (vegetable oils)
- Fish oil: 2 to 5 g (stop two weeks before surgery; continue again after surgery)
- Coenzyme Q10: 60–300 mg, in divided doses
- Vitamin E: 400–800 I.U, as *mixed tocopherols* (mixed forms of vitamin E; should be stated as such on the label)
- Alpha-lipoic acid: 600 mg (especially in people at risk of stroke)
- Milk thistle (active component: silymarin): use as tincture, three dropperfuls in a glass of water, 2 to 3 times a day in the first week after surgery
- Melatonin: 3 to 6 mg for people over age 50; 6 to 9 mg for people over age seventy; take only in the evening, within one half hour before bedtime.
- Selenium: 200 mcg
- Calcium: 1,200 mg (as calcium citrate)
- Magnesium: 500 mg
- L-carnitine: 1,000 mg, 2 to 4 times a day
- Folic acid: 800 mcg, up to 5 mg
- Vitamin B_3 (niacin): 100 mg three times a day
- Vitamin B_5 (pantothenic acid): 500 to 1,000 mg

- Phosphatidyl choline: 1 to 2 tsp
- Natural anti-inflammatory herbals, described earlier in chapter

After four to five months of using some combination of the above supplements, you may switch to an antioxidant multiple (which will be labeled as such) and continue with omega-3 supplementation indefinitely.

Coronary bypass operations and angioplasty procedures are expensive and stressful surgeries, and, more important, they do not prevent the return of coronary artery disease. Once one of these operations has been performed, focus your attention on how to keep the disease from progressing further. Low-fat, high-fiber dietary strategies have shown promise for preventing disease progression.[7] High intakes of whole grains, for example, are associated with much lower rates of ischemic heart disease,[8] Other promising strategies to help keep heart disease from advancing include some of the supplements just listed for prevention: garlic, coenzyme Q10, magnesium, selenium, soy, and vitamins C and E.[9]

In addition to these nutritional strategies, exercise and stress management can have a profound impact. Supervised cardiovascular training with heart rate monitoring may be very useful. Make arrangements before surgery to work with a special trainer or physical therapist after the operation. Also, psychological stress can worsen your vascular narrowing, or *stenosis*. Practicing relaxation techniques before, during, and after the operation is important in this regard. Finally, deep postoperative breathing is helpful because it contributes to further relaxation and moreover it decreases oxygen consumption—crucial for preventing exacerbation of any existing heart problems.

Surgery and the lungs. When surgery is done on the chest and abdomen, breathing can be limited by pain and by a malfunctioning of the diaphragm. This can result in less oxygen being available for healing. One important way to avoid these problems is to quit smoking before surgery. Stopping smoking is among the more important steps you can take to improve lung function. Doing so only 48 hours before surgery can get rid of the nicotine effect on the heart and considerably improve lung health. Stopping for 1 to 2 weeks decreases lung secretions and sputum. Stopping for 4 to 6 weeks is required to improve overall lung function on pulmonary function tests. Eight weeks free of smoking will bring the

—Antioxidants Protect Your Heart and Organs during Major Surgery—

There is now substantial evidence showing that antioxidant supplementation around the time of cardiac bypass surgery, lung transplant surgery, and other forms of surgery affecting the cardiopulmonary system can have a beneficial impact on the outcome. These surgeries can result in a major surge in oxidative stress, or excessive numbers of free radicals, which can increase the risk of various complications and even death.[10] Antioxidant supplements such as coenzyme Q10, alpha-lipoic acid, vitamins C and E, milk thistle, and melatonin prior to and after surgery can lower risk of these complications and produce better therapeutic outcomes overall.[11] The surgical technique itself is also relevant: bypass surgeries that involve coronary revascularization may require larger doses of antioxidants.[12]

During a heart attack or stroke, large numbers of harmful free radicals can be generated during a sequence of events called *ischemia-reperfusion*. Ischemia temporarily deprives the organ of oxygen, while reperfusion (a sudden influx of oxygenated blood) initiates a series of events that can exacerbate any existing tissue damage. It also occurs with surgery: surgical clamping induces ischemia, while unclamping of arteries results in reperfusion. Vitamin E, coenzyme Q10, and other antioxidant nutrients have been shown to reduce the ischemia/reperfusion injury in transplanted organs and in the heart when these supplements are taken before and after cardiac surgery.[13]

Coenzyme Q10 is a vitamin-like nutrient that appears to protect the heart from free radicals while also boosting energy production in heart cells. Your heart produces CoQ10 naturally, but as you get older it produces less; this appears to make it more vulnerable to surgical stress as well as the aerobic stress of vigorous exercise. Randomized studies of coronary bypass patients in Italy demonstrated that supplementing with coenzyme Q10 (150 mg daily, for one week before the operation) led to significantly better outcomes such as better heart function, reduced need for medication, and less oxidative stress during the procedure.[14]

Research by Dr. Franklin Rosenfeldt, head of cardiac surgical research at the Baker Institute in Melbourne, Australia, has shown that taking coenzyme Q10 before cardiac surgery improves post-operative heart function, while reducing intraoperative myocardial damage and shortening the amount of time spent in the hospital after surgery.[15] To further protect the heart against surgical stress, Dr. Rosenfeldt proposes combining coenzyme Q10 with alpha-lipoic acid, magnesium orotate, and omega 3 fatty acids before and after surgery, and integrating this strategy with a physical exercise and stress reduction program.

We believe this approach, together with a low-fat, high-fiber diet, represents a very sensible, integrative strategy for helping people prepare for and recover from the effects of cardiac or cardiopulmonary surgery. With more than 300,000 patients undergoing coronary bypass surgery and more than 400,000 getting angioplasties each year in the United States, there's a definite need for low-cost strategies that can lower your risk of life-threatening complications. Taking CoQ10 and other nutriceuticals before heading into the operating room can give you that extra resilience you need to handle the more stressful effects of these surgeries.

most cardiopulmonary benefits and decrease in symptoms (cough, shortness of breath, and sputum production). Clearly, this is an excellent self-help strategy.

Another important step is to have your physician perform spirometry, a test of lung function using a device called a spirometer. This is a kind of handheld bedside biofeedback device that measures your breathing. Spirometry can tell you whether your breathing is normal. It takes only a couple of minutes to blow into the spirometer, which can detect a problem with your breathing ability even before you do. Many physicians have a spirometer in their offices, and your hospital should give you spirometry if you're having surgery where your lungs may be affected. Taking slow deep breaths and measuring them with the spirometer can improve oxygen delivery.

A related issue that can effect how you are able to breathe after surgery is sleep apnea, a disorder in which breathing stops while you're sleeping. If you have a history of sleep apnea or heavy snoring with frequent nighttime awakenings, you may be at high risk for pulmonary problems and low oxygen levels after any surgery, especially chest surgery. Most patients with sleep apnea should not have same day surgery, but should be monitored in the hospital for 24 hours to prevent hypoxia (low oxygen); also narcotics should be avoided if possible. Please notify your doctor if you have sleep apnea or a history or snoring and daytime sleepiness. A technology called continuous positive airway pressure (CPAP) will deliver air into your airway through a specially designed nasal mask or canulas. Along with oxygen, CPAP is very helpful in the hospital and at home.

✌ Surgeries Involving the Musculoskeletal System

Any surgery that involves your joints, bones, and muscles will qualify for this category. Classic examples of surgeries that affect this system include knee surgery, hip surgery, back or spinal cord surgery, carpal tunnel surgery, and shoulder surgery. Since so many joints are included in the hands and feet, we also include both of those body parts within this category.

Many orthopedic surgery patients will benefit from taking glucosamine sulfate, chondroitin sulfate, and methylsulfonylmethane (MSM). These natural agents have been shown to promote healing of connective tissues in and around the joints. In addition, studies say supplementing with both glucosamine sulfate and chondroitin sulfate can stimulate the growth of cartilage in laboratory studies.[16] Clinical research has now clearly demonstrated the safety and efficacy of glucosamine supplementation in terms of pain relief, reduced swelling, and other symptomatic improvements following surgery.[17]

MSM is a form of organic sulfur that's naturally found in human body fluids and tissues. Although MSM originates in the ocean, most of the nutrient reaches our food supply through rainfall. As we get older, MSM levels in bodies decline, which is thought to create greater susceptibility to problems in the musculoskeletal system. The combination of glucosamine, chondroitin, and MSM can help rebuild the cartilage and stave off degenerative joint disease following any form of surgery that affects the joints.

Natural strategies for improving tissue integrity of joints, ligaments, and muscles include (dosage is daily unless otherwise specified):

- Glucosamine sulfate: 500 mg, 3 times a day
- Chondroitin sulfate: 750 mg
- MSM (methylsulfonylmethane): 1,500 to 4,500 mg
- Niacinamide (vitamin B_3 amide): 800 mg three times per day. Note: Liver enzymes must be monitored. If nausea results, then liver enzymes are elevated; however, 10 percent of the population may have elevated liver enzymes without experiencing nausea
- Vitamin B_5 (pantothenic acid): 500 mg
- Vitamin B_6: 100 mg three times a day (This treatment is especially effective for menopausal or rheumatic-type arthritis.)
- Vitamin D: 2,000 to 4,000 IU (unless you are getting out in the sun for 20 minutes a day)
- Vitamin C: 1 to 2 g (best taken in divided doses)
- Vitamin E: 400 to 1,600 IU (as mixed tocopherols)
- Selenium: 200 mcg
- Boron: 2 to 3 mg
- Calcium: 800 to 1,200 mg
- Magnesium: 500 mg
- Essential fatty acids: 2 tbsp
- Bromelain: 500 mg, 2 to 3 times a day, with food
- Prolotherapy
- Ion therapy
- Therapeutic exercise such as restorative yoga

Natural strategies for improving tissue integrity of the bones include (dosage is daily unless otherwise specified):

- Vitamin C: 2 to 3 g, in divided doses
- Vitamin B complex, as directed on the label
- Vitamin A: 20,000 IU (less in pregnancy and lactation)
- Vitamin K: 1 to 5 mg (avoid if taking blood-thinning medication)

- Vitamin B$_6$: 100 mg
- Vitamin D$_3$: 2,000 to 4,000 IU (unless you are getting out in the sun for 20 minutes a day)
- Calcium citrate: 1,000 to 1,500 mg
- Magnesium: 400 to 600 mg
- Boron: 2 to 3 mg
- Silica: 500 to 1,000 mg
- Zinc: 15 to 30 mg
- Copper: 2 to 3 mg
- DHEA: low doses (5 to 10 mg) may be especially appropriate for post-menopausal women whose serum DHEA-S levels are near or below the lower limit of normal
- Natural progesterone cream (for women)
- Gradual return to weight-bearing exercise

Recent research has shown that hypnosis combined with ideomotor movement therapy can improve rehabilitation postorthopedic surgery. Ideomotor movement therapy involves visualizing motor movements. It has long been used by professional athletes to improve performance, but can also be used for rehabilitation as well. For example, if you are stiff and have trouble getting out of bed in the morning, spending a few moments visualizing yourself getting up smoothly and effortlessly can help. In addition, establishing a passive range of motion (that is, movement without force or resistance—a wave of the arm, for example), preferably with the help of a physical therapist or massage therapist or as prescribed by your surgeon, can be helpful in the early rehabilitation process. Again, getting moving early on is crucial to improve the healing process and prevent complications.

✎ Surgeries Involving the Nervous System

Any surgery that involves your brain and nervous system will qualify for this category. The most common surgeries in this area include brain surgery and aneurysm repair. Natural strategies for bettering nervous system functioning after surgery include:

- Docosahexanoic acid (omega-3 fatty acid), from fish oil or algae: 2 to 4 g per day
- Alpha-lipoic acid: 300 mg, 3 times a day
- Phosphatidyl choline: 1 to 2 tsp
- Vitamins B$_6$: 100 to 200 mg
- Vitamins B$_{12}$: 10–50 mcg (micrograms)
- Zinc: 15 mg for women, 30 mg for men
- Ginkgo biloba: 120 to 240 mg per day in divided doses
- S-adenosylmethionine (SAM-e): 400 to 800 mg

You may take various combinations of these nutrients and botanicals—or supplements that already combine them—indefinitely to support your nervous system. A naturopathic physician or someone knowledgeable in the use of these natural agents can help you refine your choices.

❧ Surgeries Involving the Eyes

The need for eye surgery (e.g., cataract removal, radial keratotomy, and laser surgery for diabetic retinopathy) has climbed steadily in recent decades as more and more people develop cataracts, the number one cause of blindness in the world. This condition involves a thickening and clouding of the lens of the eye. As the lens becomes increasingly opaque, it is unable to transmit and focus light properly. Cataract surgery, which involves removing and replacing the lens, is among the most common types of surgery. Unfortunately, many people who have cataract surgery later suffer a detached retina or other difficulties. This is just one more reason to make sure you do everything possible to maintain good eye health before and after surgery.

Before talking about some of the natural strategies that can promote healthy vision, it's important to understand how the eyes become damaged in the first place. Exposure to ultraviolet rays and ionizing radiation leads to the formation of free radicals that damage the delicate structures within the eye. High blood pressure causes a thickening of the blood vessels inside the eye, eventually causing visual problems. Overuse of computers, lack of sleep, and excessive stress can all compromise vision over time. Lack of vegetables and other whole foods in the diet results in low levels of vitamins and phytonutrients that normally help maintain healthy vision.

High blood sugar can harm the eyes, due to reactions between glucose and proteins in the eye. This is why diabetics often develop hemorrhages in the retina and the vitreous (fluid in the eyeball), eventually producing blindness. Diabetics are also more prone to cataracts and retinopathy (damage to the retina). Research suggests that people who eat a low-fiber, low-antioxidant diet, with few vegetables and more white flour products, sugar, and other refined carbohydrate foods, are more vulnerable to eye problems.

Be aware that certain drugs, whether prescription or over the counter, can lead to eye problems as well.

As an alternative or companion to the above drugs, here are several supplements you can take to help support eye health after surgery (dosages are daily unless otherwise indicated):

- Vitamin A: 25,000 to 50,000 IU (less in pregnancy and lactation)
- Multivitamin containing high concentrations of vitamins C (1 to 3 g) and E (400 IU), as well as selenium (200 to 300 mcg daily)
- Vitamin B-complex: 100 mg 3 times daily
- Vitamin C: 2 to 6 g; a total of 12 g, in divided doses, may help relieve intraocular pressure
- Zinc: 30 to 50 mg
- Copper and manganese: 2 to 3 mg each (unless already in the multivitamin)
- Lutein: 6 mg per day (for people with macular degeneration)
- L-lysine: as directed on label, on an empty stomach; do not take with milk; take with 50 mg of vitamin B_6 and 100 mg vitamin C
- Bilberry extract: as directed on the label
- Grapeseed extract: as directed on the label
- Eyebright: as directed on the label

You may take various combinations of these nutrients and botanicals—or supplements that already combine them—indefinitely to support good eye health. But the most important period is the first three to six months after you have eye surgery.

✖ Surgeries Involving the Skin

Common surgeries involving the skin, the "largest organ of the body," include cosmetic surgery, bariatric surgery, mole removal, and, indeed, any surgery that results in substantial damage to the skin. All surgeons agree that avoiding exposure to tobacco smoke is an important way to speed up healing of the skin after plastic surgery, and most also recognize that proper nutrition is essential to healthy skin. In addition to a good diet, supplementing with specific nutrients can make a difference. For example, vitamin C helps the body create collagen, vitamin A assists in the repair of skin cells, vitamin E can reduce scarring in some wounds, and various phytonutrients can further improve your skin's vitality and ability to heal quickly. You can use these natural options to help heal the skin.

- **Healthy eating habits.** Maintain an antioxidant-boosting diet that contains plenty of vegetables, berries, cherries, and grapes on a daily basis, and consider taking a good antioxidant multiple (see chapter 4). Avoid cheese, butter, and other saturated fat sources, as well as hydrogenated fats and junk foods. Simply abstaining from sugar, white flour products, and other refined carbs can help you maintain healthier skin. These dietary habits will lead to healthier skin, less damage from sun exposure, and faster rejuvenation of your skin following surgery.

- **Hydrate.** Be sure to drink plenty of pure water—the standard advice is 6 to 8 eight-ounce glasses throughout the day—to help cleanse your body of toxins.

- **Aloe vera (internal and external).** Drink a half cup per day for one month. Aloe can also be applied externally to the wound area and may help speed up your recovery from plastic surgery.[18] Make sure your aloe product is relatively thick instead of watery—the latter consistency indicates that the aloe lacks acemannan, the active ingredient. Also make sure that the laxative compounds, called anthraquinones, have been removed from the aloe product.

- **Fish oil, flax oil, and borage oil.** Take 1 to 2 teaspoons per day, with food. These oils can help balance the inflammatory systems of the body and this, in turn, supports better skin health and better tissue repair. (Remember to avoid taking these oils for one week prior to surgery and on the day of surgery.)

- **Skin creams containing antioxidants.** Pharmaceutical-grade ingredients, including tretinoin (retin-A, a derivative of vitamin A) and topical vitamin C, have been effective in speeding up healing after cosmetic surgery and improving the appearance of damaged skin.[19] Topical vitamin E cream can also help reduce scarring in some wound situations, though the results have been inconsistent. (Caution: Do not use tretinoin if you're also using Saint-John's-wort, as this may result in a photosensitivity reaction.) Herbal skin creams containing calendula, jojoba oil, or rosehip oil may help improve the elasticity of the skin.

- **Comfrey salve (topical).** Apply salve to wound area three to four times a day; clean wound area thoroughly before applying the salve. Made from the roots of fresh comfrey, the salve is used to sooth and heal inflamed tissues, and to help reduce swelling and pain. Many comfrey salve preparations also contain vitamin E and lavender oil to further soften the skin and combat skin irritation.

- **Detoxification strategies.** Regular consumption of broccoli sprouts will accelerate the detoxification process, as will certain herbs that should be used under the direction of a naturopathic doctor or herbalist (e.g., dandelion, milk thistle).

- **Sauna therapy.** Saunas once a day during the cleansing period will open the pores of the skin and release toxins that can impede healing.

- **Aerobic exercise.** Try to exercise at least a half hour each session, three to five times a week. Exercise enhances blood flow and thereby helps deliver more nutrients to your skin. Sweating during vigorous exercise can further accelerate the removal of toxins.

- **Hormone balancing.** This requires testing and consultation with an allopathic or naturopathic physician or other health care professional who understands hormonal balancing. The key hormones of interest are growth hormone, estrogens, testosterone, DHEA, and cortisol.

❧ Concerns and Caveats for Special Circumstances

Whenever you face surgery, ask yourself whether there's anything about your personal health history that could put you more at risk for complications after surgery or problems that could prevent a smooth recovery. We have compiled a list of some of the more common concerns and caveats for people in specific circumstances.

Surgeries for pediatric patients. Most of the recommendations and doses in this book are for adult surgery patients. Please consult with your pediatric surgeon or pediatrician before giving any of the supplements to children. However, many of the mind-body techniques such as imagery, relaxation, and hypnosis have been successfully used with children. Manual therapies such as massage and osteopathic manipulation are also known to be safe and effective. Spiritual support with prayer has been shown to be helpful for many medical and surgical outcomes. This type of support is quite safe to use with kids.

Surgery during pregnancy and breast-feeding. Many of the herbs and supplements included in this book are not known to be safe to take during pregnancy and breast-feeding. In particular, high doses of vitamin A can be harmful to the developing child. Please consult your ob-gyn prior to using any of those therapies. Most body-mind therapies have been studies and successfully used in pregnancy, labor, and surgery. Hypnosis (using glove anesthesia and dissociation), relaxation, and imagery are especially useful. These techniques use suggestions to spread a numbing sensation or promote a distraction from pain. Acupuncture has been well studied in pregnancy and is helpful for decreasing pain and nausea. Massage can be useful, as can spiritual support. With breast-feeding it is best to put off elective surgery until you've stopped. For nonelective surgeries, local or regional anesthesia (epidural or spinal) will have the least effect on the baby. General anesthesia, which requires large doses of narcotics, may enter the breast milk and necessitate pumping and dumping of the milk for 6 to 24 hours, depending on dose, age of the infant, and length of surgery.

Surgeries for people with cancer. A crucial concern for cancer patients is that surgery creates inflammation, which in turn ups the level of growth factors in the blood. These growth factors may stimulate the proliferation of residual cancer cells or distant metastases. For example, animal studies have shown that surgical trauma results in circulating growth factors that are needed for tissue regeneration around the surgical wound; however, these same growth factors were also shown to stimulate the growth of cancer cells located elsewhere in the body.[20] One of the great benefits of fish oil supplementation before and after surgery is that it can help temper the inflammatory response that gives way to excessive growth factor production.[21] Fish oil also kills cancer cells directly and can help limit the tendency toward chronic inflammation that leads to runaway weight loss in so many cancer patients.[22]

❧❧❧

ELLEN'S STORY: HEALING FROM BREAST CANCER SURGERY

The following is told in the first person by Ellen, a breast cancer patient.

On Halloween day, 2002, I was diagnosed with stage 2 breast cancer. The tumor was large—a little over 3 centimeters in diameter—and during surgery it was determined that cancer had spread into the lymphatic and vascular systems. I went on to receive 6 months of chemotherapy. During this time, a genetic test showed that I was a carrier of a genetic mutation (BRCA II), which placed me at high risk of recurring breast cancer in either breast, as well as a substantial risk of ovarian cancer. I opted for a bilateral mastectomy and oophrectomy (removal of the ovaries).

While at a yoga class, I met a man with advanced melanoma, who referred me to Mark Mead for health coaching and information about tissue repair. The man said that Mark's coaching had transformed his quality of life for the better, and that his speedy recovery from surgery had astonished his surgeon and physical therapist.

Mark and I then laid out a comprehensive plan for nutrition, meditation, sleep management, and supplements to enhance recovery and build disease resistance. I have been on this plan for three years. To my amazement and delight, I have more energy and am in better physical shape than before the onset of cancer—despite creeping middle age (I am forty-eight years old).

Between my lumpectomy, oophrectomy, mastectomy, and breast reconstruction, I have had six surgeries to date. After the last surgery, the area of the incision became infected, and a patch of skin died, leaving a one-inch triangle of raw, inflamed flesh. The area was slow to heal, and my surgeon did not offer any treatment that would speed up the recovery. Two months after surgery, the area was still an open wound, and it seemed that recovery had stopped.

At this point, I contacted Mark again, to ask for his suggestions in using nutrition and other complementary therapies for healing. Mark shared research showing the wound-healing benefits of certain supplements, such as higher doses of vitamin C, zinc, and gotu kola, and high-quality fish oil. He also convinced me to try two topical creams, aloe vera and calendula, both of which I applied alternately morning and night.

The tissues seemed to heal and close up almost overnight. Within 10 days, a film of new skin had formed on the area, and the bleeding and oozing stopped. I am continuing the treatment, hoping that in two months the skin will be thick and resistant enough to withstand another surgery—hopefully my last.

<hr />

Surgery and allergies. Most patients know to tell their doctor if they're allergic to medication. But it's also important to alert your physician to any food or latex allergies. If you will be hospitalized and the hospital will be providing food, make sure you aren't given anything that could trigger a reaction. Be particularly careful with latex—many medical devices and gloves contain latex, which could be dangerous if they're used inadvertently around a patient who's allergic.

Surgery and steroid medication. It is critically important to notify your physician if you've taken steroids like prednisone (at a minimum, 5 mg per day for one week) in the preceding nine months. This dose could suppress your adrenal gland. If your doctor is alerted, he can give you appropriate adrenal support.

Note that inhaled steroids do not pose a problem in this context.

—Surgery, High Blood Sugar, and Insulin—

Blood sugar levels rise almost immediately after a surgery begins. The more aggressive or invasive the procedure, the greater the elevation in blood sugar. For example, glucose levels rise dramatically and often remain elevated for more than 24 hours after heart surgery.

Why does this occur? One reason is that the stress hormones that start rising with surgery—cortisol, adrenaline, and others—tend to stimulate the production of glucose from the liver. At the same time, the muscles and other tissues take up less glucose, apparently due to the problem known as *insulin resistance*. Insulin is the hormone that helps usher glucose into your body cells. Insulin resistance is the condition in which the hormone is not being utilized by your body cells; this invariably results in high blood sugar levels.

When your blood sugar swings up and down, you are at greater risk of infection and heart attack. If you're a diabetic, be sure that you have an EKG in order to determine whether you have a fast heart rate or lack of variability. You should also have your blood pressure checked while standing, as this provides yet another indicator for the functionality of your autonomic nervous system.

There is little doubt that better blood sugar control results in better wound healing. This has been clearly shown in people with diabetes.[23] Diabetic complications such as foot infections and poor wound healing are significantly fewer with better control of blood sugar.[24] By maintaining the blood sugar level at less than 200 mg/dL, wound healing happens more smoothly.[25]

One possible way to reduce the problem of insulin resistance after surgery is to "carbo load"—consume more pasta and other carbohydrate-rich foods before the operation, and avoid prolonged fasting.[26] It is possible that fasting before surgery does contribute to insulin resistance after surgery. However, fasting for at least eight hours will be necessary to safely administer anesthesia in most cases.

Lastly, it is possible that supplementation with chromium and carnosine will affect blood sugar metabolism and therefore further help improve the wound healing in diabetics or people who have recently undergone major surgery. The trace element chromium improves both blood sugar control and insulin sensitivity in people with diabetes.[27] Carnosine blocks glycation, one of the main mechanisms that links blood sugar to poor wound healing.[28] The research to date also suggests that antioxidant supplements like alpha-lipoic acid and vitamins C and E can also counteract glycation and improve wound healing even when blood sugar levels are relatively high.

A low-fat, high-fiber diet and regular exercise can further reduce insulin resistance and improve blood sugar control. Avoid sugar, white flour products, and other refined foods before, during, and immediately after surgery in order to lower your risk of infection and mortality. Finally, certain diabetic medications should be stopped or monitored carefully in order to prevent blood sugar imbalances. Your surgeon may want to use insulin briefly around the time of surgery to optimize glucose control—be sure that your physicians and nurses know if you're a diabetic or borderline diabetic so that blood sugars can be monitored and medications adjusted accordingly.

❦ Core Nutrition for Long-Range Recovery

When you think about bolstering your body's ability to mend after surgery, it's important to consider both the short term and the long term. In chapters 6 and 7, we addressed the short term—the various issues that can affect your repair and recovery within the first few months of surgery. In general, the first 2 weeks after surgery are the pivotal time for managing pain and inflammation, and for dealing with the more serious risks associated with major surgery. It is also a critical period for promoting tissue repair through optimal nutrition and other strategies. But healing can go on for a very long time. Older people (over age forty) who had received multiple operations may continue to feel weak, fatigued, or "below par" for many months. In some cases, the aftereffects of surgery can last for years.

Remember that major surgery requires extensive tissue repair and can deplete the body of vital resources. As part of your plan for long-range recovery, you should of course try to maintain a healthy diet, regular exercise, and stress management. Dietary considerations may be especially important in the case of people undergoing surgery for heart problems, kidney problems, and digestive and gastrointestinal problems. In general, try to maintain the following dietary principles.

- **High fiber, low sugar.** Consume primarily whole grains, legumes, and vegetables; avoid white flour products and artificial sweeteners.

- **Low-fat diet, avoiding saturated fats in particular.** Minimize intake of red meats, poultry, and fatty dairy products; use olive oil, canola oil, rice kernel oil, and coconut oil. Avoid hydrogenated oils (margarine, vegetable shortenings, imitation butter spreads, and most commercial peanut butters) and oxidized fats (barbequed meats, deep fried foods, fast food, and ghee).

- **Calorie percentages.** Consume a diet made up of 60 to 70 percent complex carbohydrates, 15 to 20 percent protein, 15 to 20 percent fat (along with omega-3 supplementation).

- **Consider cleansing periodically.** Use a vegetarian cleansing diet that emphasizes more water and vegetable juices, small portions of food, plus sizable amounts of alfalfa sprouts, garlic, scallions, watercress, apple, celery, berries, and cherries.

In addition to these dietary principles, we recommend that you explore the use of the following "multiples" for the long term, each of which may provide a better fit for your particular circumstances.

1. **Multivitamin-mineral complex: for general nutritional support.**
Pollution, toxins, stress, aging, illness, and medical treatments can greatly increase the body's nutritional needs, in essence creating "conditional deficiencies." As far back as 1936, a congressional commission reported on the floor of the Senate that the typical U.S. diet failed to provide adequate minerals to maintain good health. Since that time, modern farming techniques have continued to erode the nutritional quality of our food supply. The chemicals used in fertilizers, pesticides, and herbicides have helped produce foodstuffs in ever more quantity, but at the expense of topsoil minerals. Organically grown foods not only contain more nutrients but also fewer pollutants. In the June 2002 issue of the *Journal of the American Medical Association,* medical researchers from several leading research institutions recommended that all North Americans take a multivitamin in order to ensure nutritional sufficiency.

One of the main advantages of taking a multinutrient supplement is that you can take advantage of *synergisms* or cooperative relationships between the different nutrients. This means that combining one or more of the nutrients results in a greater degree of benefit than if the nutrients were used in isolation. When a synergism exists between two or more nutrients, we mean that the combination results in better absorption and assimilation of the nutrients. Alternatively, the synergism may bring certain physiologic benefits, such as enhanced antioxidant protection or immune responsiveness. Many of these nutritional preparations are designed with synergisms in mind.

Look for a balanced and fully absorbable multinutrient supplement derived from natural sources, ideally one that includes some plant-derived ingredients. The preparation should satisfy the full daily requirements for: niacin, folic acid, pantothenic acid, vitamin B_1, vitamin B_2, vitamin B_6, vitamin B_{12}, vitamin C, vitamin E, copper, chromium, zinc, selenium, and manganese. Multiples should always be taken with food, preferably just before you eat a balanced or mixed meal. If your diet is replete with whole grains, legumes, fruits, and vegetables, you can usually take half of the recommended dose of a multiple and still derive ample benefit.

2. **Antioxidant multiple: for people over age forty who have undergone major surgery or who have a family history of cancer.** A variety of factors can generate free radicals, including inflammation, dietary fats, and pollutants such as tobacco smoke and chemicals. As we get older, our ability to resist the damaging effects of free radicals declines. The antioxidants in your body and diet are necessary in adequate quantities to counter the destructive impact of these highly reactive molecules. Look for a balanced antioxidant formula that contains three or more of the following antioxidant factors: alpha-lipoic acid, coenzyme Q10, bilberry extract, lycopene, L-carnitine, broccoli extract (flavonones), N-acetyl cysteine (NAC), green tea catechins, and grapeseed extract (proanthocyanidins). These antioxidants work within your body at the molecular level; they enter the normally impregnable cell and attach themselves to any free radical found within the cell. This gives you a higher level of protection.

Antioxidant multiples can be taken daily or on days when you plan to be engaged in vigorous aerobic exercise. If you are recovering from disease, showing signs of inflammation, or not maintaining a high intake of fruits and vegetables, then consider taking an antioxidant more frequently.

3. **Omega-3 fatty acids: for people who have consumed a significant amount of meats, dairy products, and refined carbohydrate foods for many years**. Back in prehistoric times, the human diet was well en-

dowed with omega-3 fatty acids. Whether our food came from wild game or plants, we consumed plenty of omega-3s on a daily basis. These dietary habits would have strongly supported the body's ability to combat chronic inflammation, since omega-3 fats provide the raw materials for keeping these inner fires in check. Today, however, modern farming has brought about a loss in genetic diversity in the food supply, so that most food products (with the exception of fatty fish) contain little or no omega-3 fatty acids. Here in the United States, it is estimated that the average consumption of omega-3 fatty acids is *10 to 20 times lower* than it was in the past.[29] It's likely that this lack of dietary omega-3 fats plays a major role in heart disease, arthritis, and many other chronic inflammatory problems that plague our society today.[30]

To bolster your body's anti-inflammatory potential before and after surgery, we recommend using an omega-3 supplement on a daily basis. For the first 3 months, use an omega-3 supplement that is either pure EPA or very high in EPA, then switch for 3 more months to a fish oil preparation balanced in both EPA and DHA. Finally, for long-range consumption, try to find an omega-3 supplement that contains EPA, DHA, and borage oil.

Note: Omega-3 fatty acids may initially be consumed in larger quantity (4 to 6 grams per day) if you are losing weight after major surgery. This higher dose also has been shown to help preserve kidney function (glomerular filtration rate) due to cyclosporine treatment.[31] After one month, the dosage can be reduced to 1 to 3 grams per day, depending on your body weight and on whether you still show signs of inflammation. Remember that you want to stop taking fish oil at least one week before surgery and check with your physician if you're taking blood-thinning medications.

4. **Anti-inflammatory multiple: for people who have undergone major surgery and have ongoing inflammatory tendencies**. Some people continue to have joint and muscle pain and other inflammatory symptoms long after their surgery. The following signs and symptoms may indicate some degree of inflammatory imbalance: pain and stiffness

in the morning, red eyes, swollen ankles, dry skin, chronically runny nose, allergies, and chronically impacted ear wax. The underlying inflammatory dysfunction can predispose you to hay fever, hives, asthma, arthritis, colitis, inflammatory bowel syndrome, lupus erythematosis, multiple sclerosis, and seborrheic dermatitis.

If you show signs of ongoing inflammation, even with fish oil supplementation, you might benefit from a multiple that contains more vitamin E and selenium, as well as curcumin, boswellia, holy basil, quercetin, green tea, and bromelain. These herbal agents will nicely complement the effects of the omega-3 fatty acids. You don't have to take them every day, but note that they can help reduce your dependency on selective COX-2 inhibitors that have recently been linked with higher rates of heart attack.

In this chapter, we have explored a variety of strategies that can be applied to specific surgical scenarios. There are many factors to take into account when designing an approach that is appropriate for you, given your history, biochemical individuality, and medical circumstances. We urge you to consult with qualified health care professionals when attempting to incorporate these strategies into your own self-care plan before, during, and after surgery.

9

Life after the Knife

Time heals all wounds.

—Anon

*I always try to get patients to see
standard medical treatment—such as
radiation, chemotherapy, and surgery—
as energy that can heal them. They buy
time during which I can help the
patient find the will to live, change,
and heal. Many of the disagreements
over the worth of alternate therapies
arise because some people heal
themselves no matter what external
aides they choose, as long as they have
hope and some control over the therapy.
I support them as long as a patient has
chosen them with a positive conviction,
not out of fear.*

—Bernie Siegel, MD,
Love, Medicine, and Miracles

As physicians and health care practitioners working in the area of integrative medicine, we have a tremendous responsibility. After all, many people come to us for guidance around the time of surgery and other major medical events. Our task is not simply to help them "get through" surgery, but to do so as smoothly and rapidly as possible. Our goal is not just to ensure recovery, but to promote an *optimal* recovery—one that leads to better health and better functioning for the long term. If we don't impress upon them the value of improving their nutrition, exercise habits, sleep hygiene, and other aspects of self-care, chances are that they will maintain their old habits and their recovery will be less than optimal.

In the preceding chapters, we identified a treasure trove of natural agents and other tools for enhancing your ability to repair your tissues after surgery and speed up your recovery. Many of these tools can also be used to support your *long-range* recovery after surgery. For example, we mentioned a number of factors that influence the production of inflammatory chemicals in the body.

One of the long-range issues a patient may face is chronic, low-level inflammation. Remember that surgery itself can unleash a powerful wave of chronic inflammation in the body, but this inflammation only continues if the patient has an inappropriate diet and lifestyle habits. Chronic inflammation can impede healing and promote a variety of health problems that can necessitate the need for further surgery.

Among the diet and lifestyle habits that can greatly help keep chronic inflammation in check, thereby bolstering your rapid repair potential, are the following:

- **Eating well is key.** The typical U.S. diet lacks fruits and vegetables and contains excessive amounts of meat, dairy, and refined carbohydrate foods. This kind of diet may be the perfect recipe for supporting chronic pain, chronic inflammation, and inflammation-related diseases.[1] Regular consumption of saturated fat, animal protein, and refined carbohydrate foods—white flour products and artificial sweeteners, candy and sugary beverages—leads to a variety of biochemical changes that cause the body to generate more inflammation. Try to limit their consumption and instead eat more fiber. Simply by eating a whole-foods, vegetable-based diet, you can avoid fanning those fires within.

- **Favor those fish fats.** The omega-6 fatty acids in our foods—mostly in vegetable oils, red meat, poultry, and dairy products—all promote inflammation in our bodies. Omega-3 fatty acids have the opposite effect, and yet most Americans consume only a tiny fraction of the omega-3 fats they need for optimal health and inflammatory control. Fish oil supplements are the most reliable source of omega-3 fats in terms of controlling inflammation. As noted earlier in the book, make sure you get a supplement that is processed with molecular distillation under oxygen-free conditions; these two factors result in a pure product that does not contain any oxidized fats.

- **Lay off the "hydrog."** The hydrogenated oils, or "trans fats," we get from margarine and many processed foods provide powerful fuel for inflammation. Like saturated fats, the hydrogenated fats will promote a rise in oxidized LDL, the so-called bad cholesterol, which tends to further amplify the inflammatory process. As much as possible, try to avoid these artificial sources of fat in your daily diet.

- **Exercise in moderation.** Regular exercise is good for your health and for inflammatory control, but too much strenuous exercise will increase your inflammatory tendencies. The trick is to find a rhythm whereby you exercise without strain on a regular basis, several times a week if possible. Give your body time to build up to a level of exertion, and give it time to recover after a vigorous workout before you exercise again. (Be sure to read our exercise tips for postoperative recovery in chapter 6.) An antioxidant-rich diet and supplement plan will help your body deal with the more stressful effects of intensive exercise training.

- **Watch the wine and spirits.** Hard alcohol and excessive imbibing in general can weaken the body's anti-inflammatory mechanisms, thereby increasing your tendency to become chronically inflamed. With the exception of the occasional glass of red wine or beer, try to stay away from alcohol. With limited use of alcohol, you can always enjoy a different kind of "happy hour." This is particularly important in the first few months after surgery.

- **Steer clear of smoke and pollution.** Habitual smoking promotes low-level inflammation in the lungs. Smoking is also a major source of free radicals, which help perpetuate chronic inflammation. But air pollution in general—whether from automotive exhaust, ozone, or industrial emissions—promotes inflammatory reactions in the body. Try to avoid breathing in too much polluted air, whether from indoor or outdoor sources (use air filters, plants, and other strategies). And steer clear of areas where people are smoking. If you're a smoker and having trouble kicking the habit, try harder—with acupuncture, herbal and nicotine gum, and even self-hypnosis if need be.

- **Keep allergies and infections under control.** Allergies and infections can be a source of chronic inflammation. Many of these problems are hidden or below the medical radar, either because they do not cause immediate problems (e.g., delayed allergic reactions) or because you become accustomed to the discomfort. Yeast and parasitic infections are common examples of infections that often go untreated until they are far advanced. Consult with medical experts if you suspect your body may be harboring either or both of these problems.

- **Trim that body fat.** Body fat is a source of natural chemicals that can promote chronic inflammation. This is why overweight people are prone to all kinds of inflammatory problems. At the same time, when you lose weight, your tendency to become and remain inflamed decreases. Keep in mind that if you're overweight, you will need more fish oil to eventually displace all the bad fats from your cell membranes.

After you've recovered from your surgery, keep your body's anti-inflammatory and antioxidant power as strong as possible. By doing so, you'll lower your risk of developing degenerative diseases later on, and you will reduce your need for anti-inflammatory drugs. Having a test called the high-sensitivity C-reactive protein (CRP) can help you determine whether you have chronic inflammation and need to take aggressive measures such as those outlined in this book. Any prolonged elevation of your CRP, as well as any prolonged elevation of oxidative stress indicators (such as oxidized LDL), is a perfectly good reason to clean up your act and follow the guidelines mentioned above. If you do return to surgery again, you'll be in much better shape to handle the treatment.

Surgery for most people is an unexpected and often unwelcome event. No one is happy to hear, "I'm afraid you will need surgery for . . ." And yet, in most cases, it is a necessary healing and sometimes lifesaving process. The suffering you may experience from the procedure often has little to do with side effects or even pain, but rather from the meaning you place on the experience. If you see yourself as singled out and helpless, and the process as pointless and interminable, you will undoubtedly suffer more.

We hope this book has shown you that you're not alone, and that there are many ways to find support from the universe. You are far from helpless when it comes to healing from even the most drastic procedures. Our first suggestion to this end is to voice out loud the following affirmation:

"I am fully supported in my health and healing. The choices I make daily, the ways I choose to live my life—all make a major difference in my ability to heal. Every moment of every day, I make choices that can positively influence my personal well-being."

This affirmation may empower you to be more attentive toward the choices that have become unconscious, health-negating habits over the years. In other words, you may not be consciously aware of how these choices affect you in the moment or later on, but you make them nonetheless. Every time you choose a food to eat, an exercise to perform, or a way of responding to some situation in the high-pressure arena of life, you are influencing your health in subtle and diverse ways.

Second, remember that surgery and recovery have a distinct repair and recovery phase. A few months from now, this stress will be all behind you and you can move on to greater functioning and well-being. Although the challenges of postoperative recovery can at times seem overwhelming, they will eventually pass.

Third and last, your injury or illness does have meaning. And yet it is up to you to discover what that meaning is. Perhaps it is an insight into how you want to spend your free time, or a new life path you would like to take. Perhaps it is a lesson about dietary and lifestyle choices you want to embrace. Perhaps it will be an opportunity to learn about trust, creativity, and personal power. Perhaps the experience of injury or illness may inspire you to help another, reconnect to family or friends or to a higher power.

Many of our patients tell us that their surgical experience—if it was an arduous or challenging one—became an opportunity for these kinds of personal reflection. Those who had the surgery in response to a physical ailment or disease often use the surgery as an opportunity for reorienting their lives in totally unexpected and expansive ways.

❧

NADINE'S SURGERY AS A TURNING POINT

When I met Nadine in the emergency room, I found her suffering from a large vulvar abscess. Technically, an abscess is a localized collection of pus in part of the body, usually formed because of an infection and surrounded by an inflamed area that can be very painful to the touch. Nadine had a high fever and low blood pressure, and her blood sugar levels were extremely high due to her diabetes. She was twenty-nine years old, weighed 245 pounds, and looked very sick. The abscess turned out to be a life-threatening bacterial infection, and I knew she would likely end up in the ICU if she survived. This is not what I consider to be the ideal situation for surgery, with no time for nutritional preparation or stress management training— but there was also no time to lose. I started her on antibiotics and rushed her to the operating room to remove the abscess.

Nadine did survive, and after some days in the ICU on a ventilator her infection subsided. We corrected her metabolic problems and got her blood sugar levels back to normal. Once she was on the regular hospital service, we had a long talk about her close call. The crisis had really shaken her up. She told me she never wanted to feel that way again. I told her there were many ways she could work to transform her health—that with diet, exercise, and mind-body care she could improve the control of her diabetes, improve her immune function, and decrease her risk of infection.

Our conversation became a powerful catalyst for change: Nadine immediately set to work by focusing on all the ways she could improve her nutrition. She began by buying some whole-foods-based cookbooks and clearing out all the refined and overly processed foods from her kitchen. She got serious about her fitness as well, committing to 4 days of cycling and brisk walking each week. She embraced with gusto a stricter diet and began using specific supplements to improve her blood sugar, enhance immunity, and keep inflammation and infections at bay. In addition, she received hydrotherapy treatments and careful wound care. Within a very short period, her wound had healed up completely.

The surgery gave Nadine a new lease on life. In the last four years she has lost thirty-five pounds, and she says her energy levels have never been better. I've only had the pleasure of seeing her in the office—no more visits to the ER. Sometimes you may not have the opportunity to do all you would like before surgery, but there's still much that can be done to aid repair in the postoperative period.

—EGM

Along these lines, you might consider asking the following basic questions after your surgery: How can I reorient my daily life so that I maintain health and wellness today and for the rest of my life? How can I reclaim my body's self-healing wisdom? How can I recover a sense of lightness and vitality that makes me want to continue taking good care of myself? These are the kinds of questions that will lead you to discover a rhythm to your daily life in which it becomes easier to eat well, enjoy life, and stay healthy on an ongoing basis.

What we're suggesting is that you use your experience of surgery to motivate yourself in the direction of a health-promoting diet and lifestyle for the long term. This may simply mean taking what you did to bolster your postoperative recovery and allowing this to carry over to your everyday existence. A long-range view is required to make this happen. Most people stop woefully short in their quest for health by satisfying themselves with a quick-fix solution rather than aspiring to the deeper levels of vitality and resilience that lead to long-range well-being. With a diet and lifestyle such as the one we've outlined above and in earlier chapters, you can realize this greater level of vitality and lower the risk of serious degeneration for the future.

Whether your motivation is to prevent disease or reverse cellular damage and degeneration, all the practical solutions have one thing in common: a commitment to discovering the proper balance within yourself in order to maintain healthy patterns of daily living. You need to find the right balance of foods, supplements, and activities that work for you on a day-to-day basis. Your personal vision of health will continue to evolve as you reclaim, on an experiential level, an authentic level of fitness—a deeper sense of wellness, a more complete level of functioning that encompasses both body and mind, a greater sense of engagement with your own life and with the community of people around you.

You now have numerous tools for enhancing wound healing, the natural process of repair that occurs when your body tissues are injured. But the challenges of healing often take us beyond the pragmatic and concrete, beyond the nuts and bolts of tending to the complex needs of our bodies. Surgery can be a harmonious and uneventful experience, but it can also be a very taxing, dramatic, and difficult experience. It can challenge you to live more sanely and salubriously, with greater appreciation for what it means to have a fully functioning body. We hope that your surgery will serve as a catalyst for taking greater responsibility for your personal growth and well-being. Finally, we hope that with the information presented in this handbook, you will be able to see yourself as one of many people who are now empowered to facilitate their body's innate healing wisdom, and that you will actively continue to support your total being on its healing journey.

❧The Master Table for Rapid Repair and Recovery

Here is an overview of what steps to take during each phase of the healing process. Use it as a road map to navigate through your recovery program, but please refer to earlier chapters for specific details regarding the implementation of these suggestions and for additional options that may be beneficial for your particular situation.

I. *Preparation for Surgery (Preoperative Phase)*	
Fortifying Your Healing Resources (4 to 8 Weeks Prior to Surgery)	
Nutritional Care	Power Healing Drink (see page 73)
	Whole foods, vegetable-rich diet (moderate protein, low fat)
	Omega-3 supplement (EPA/DHA combination, 2 to 4 g/day)*
	Vitamin C (500 to 3,000 mg/day)
	Balanced multivitamin

Mind-Body Care	Learn relaxation techniques
	Listen to relaxation or self-hypnosis tapes
	Establish your support team (or network), and gather information about your surgery

Body-Centered Care	Consider massage for relaxation
	Regular aerobic exercise and muscle toning
	Consider acupuncture or acupressure

| **Lifestyle** | Stop smoking, limit alcohol intake |

*Note: Stop taking the omega-3 supplement 7 days before surgery. Decrease your intake of vitamin C to 500 mg 3 days before surgery.

2. *Immediate Postsurgery (Phases 1 and 2 of the Healing Process)*

Wound-Sealing Phase (Days 1 to 5 after Surgery)
and
Inflammatory Phase (Days 1 to 21 after Surgery)

Nutritional Care	Power Healing Drink
	Liquid diet or easily digestible diet, plus berries, grapes, cherries
	Balanced multivitamin
	Antioxidant multiple
	Lactobacillus (or balanced probiotic supplement)*
	Anti-inflammatory options:

(a) Nutriceuticals: buffered vitamin C (1 to 5 g/day), vitamin E (mixed tocopherols, 400 to 600 IU/day), selenium (150 to 250/day), alpha-lipoic acid (300 mg 3×/day), N-acetyl cysteine (500 to 1,000 mg), taurine (500 mg 3×/day), GLA (500 to 1,000 mg/day), and omega-3 (either fish oil or pure EPA, 1 to 3 g/day)*

(b) Herbals: curcumin, boswellia, bromelain, and holy basil (for dosages, see Table 7.3, page 180).

Caution: if using anti-inflammatory medication, avoid combining it with high doses of fish oil, vitamin E, ginkgo, garlic, and other blood-thinning supplements listed in Table 8.1, page 201.

Mind-Body Care	Practice deep breathing with incentive spirometry
	Continue to use self-hypnosis healing tapes
	Connect with family and friends
Body-Centered Care	Ice and elevation for swelling as is appropriate
	Light lymph-mobilizing Swedish-type massage or gentle osteopathic manipulative therapy
	Walking and gentle range-of-motion exercises
	Consider acupuncture or acupressure
Lifestyle	Continue to avoid tobacco and alcohol
	Get plenty of rest and extra sleep

*Note: This probiotic supplement is especially valuable for anyone who has received antibiotics during or after his/her surgery. Most probiotics contain a variety of "healthy" bacterial cultures that will boost your intestinal integrity and improve digestion.

3. *Short-Term Healing Postsurgery (Phase 3 of the Healing Process)*

Tissue-Building Phase (Days 4 to 90)

Nutritional Care	Power Healing Drink
	Whole foods, vegetable- and protein-rich diet (high fiber, mildly low fat)
	Fish oil or DHA/EPA (1 to 4 gm/day)
	Antioxidant-rich multiple
	Lactobacillus (or balanced probiotic supplement)
	Tissue-building options:

(a) Nutriceuticals: vitamin C (1 to 3g/day), antioxidant multiple (should contain alpha-lipoic acid and phytonutrients such as bioflavonoids, grapeseed extract, berry extracts, and green tea), L-glutamine (500 to 5,000 mg/day), glucosamine sulfate (500 mg 3×/day), L-arginine (10 to 20 g/day),* MSM (1g 2×/day), and gotu kola (400 mg capsule, 3×/day)

(b) Botanicals: curcumin (400 mg 3×/day), bromelain (500 mg 3×/day), and boswellia (also b/Boswellin; 500 mg 3×/day); aloe vera concentrate (3 tbs to a full cup, daily)

	Avoid: sweets, refined carbohydrates, hydrogenated fats, omega-6-rich oils (e.g., corn oil, safflower oil, sunflower oil), fatty meats, and dairy products
Mind-Body Care	Use support to integrate surgical outcomes into meaningful and healthy lifestyle
	Continue regular practice of relaxation
Body-Centered Care	Physical therapy: as directed by your physician
	Gentle stretching
	Gradual increase to moderate level of exercise in the fat-burn heart rate range
	Limit lifting to 15 lbs until 6 weeks for major surgery
	After 6 weeks, okay to work on strengthening core with Pilates
Lifestyle	Continue to avoid tobacco and passive smoke
	Maintain a balance between rest and activity
	Maintain healthy sleep habits

---

*Note: Avoid supplementing with arginine (or L-arginine) if you have just undergone surgery as part of cancer treatment.

4. Long-Term Healing Postsurgery
(Phase 4 of the Healing Process)

Matrix-Maturing Phase (3 Months to 3 Years)

Nutritional Care	Power Healing Drink
	Whole foods, vegetable-rich diet (high fiber, moderate protein, mildly low fat)
	High-quality fish oil (1 g/day) plus GLA (50 mg)*
	Balanced multivitamin

   Note: The specific selection and combination of these factors will vary depending on the situation, as we address in chapter 8.

Mind-Body Care	Practice regular relaxation and mindfulness in daily life
Body-Centered Care	Feel free to intensify your workout routine
Lifestyle	Continue to avoid tobacco and passive smoke
	Maintain a balance between rest and activity
	Maintain healthy sleep habits

---

*Note: GLA is helpful in balancing the metabolism of omega-3 fats (EPA/DHA) from fish oil. Nonetheless, GLA itself can become a proinflammatory factor unless balanced by a high-quality omega-3 supplement. Therefore, do not use GLA supplements (e.g., borage and evening primrose oil) long term without balancing them with at least 20 times more EPA/DHA from fish oil (e.g., 50 mg GLA to 1,000 mg fish oil per day).

❦Appendix A
Nutriceutical and Botanical Supplement Sources

Below are 27 specific supplement types with brand names and company sources. Our clinical experience suggests that these are reliable products and companies. These may be available at your local health food store, through the Internet (a list of Web sites follows), or directly from the companies themselves.

❦ Green Foods (Superfood Concentrates)

Green Vibrance—by Vibrant Health
Berry Green—by New Chapter
Best of Greens—by Platinum Health Products
Green Defense—by Jarrow
Greens+—by Greens+

❦ Whey Protein

Whey To Go—by Solgar
365 Whey Protein—by Whole Foods

Spiru-Tein Whey—by Nature's Plus
Whey Protein—by Jarrow
Whey to Health—by Source Naturals
Show-Me-The-Whey—by Triangle Nutrition

∾ Omega-3 Fatty Acids

Fish Oil

Ultimate Omega, EPA, and EPA Xtra (pills or liquid)—by Nordic Naturals

RxOmega-3 Factors (pills or liquid)—by Natural Factors

Finest Fish Oil Liquid Omega-3, or Super Omega-3 Fish Oils (pills)—Carlson Laboratories

Flax Oil, Liquid Preferred (Takes 14 Capsules to Equal 1 Tablespoon of Liquid)—Some Companies/Sources for This Supplement

Spectrum, Barlean's, Whole Foods

Ground Flaxseed Brands

Ground Premium Flax—by Spectrum Organic Products
FiproFlax—by Health From The Sun
Forti-Flax—by Barlean's

∾ Borage Oil/Evening Primrose (As Well As Pure GLA Supplements)

Spectrum (organic EPO)
Barlean's (organic EPO)
Whole Foods (organic EPO), regular borage

❧ Combination Omega 3s and 6s

Complete Omega 3-6-9 (pills or liquid)—by Nordic Naturals

RxOmega-3 Factors Fish Oil Concentrate with Evening Primrose & Flaxseed Oils (pills)—by Natural Factors

❧ Anti-inflammatory Multiple

Zyflamend—by New Chapter

Inflama-Rest—by Source Naturals

Herbal Ease—by Viable Herbal Solutions

Itis-Care—by Narula Research

❧ Probiotics

Jarro-Dophilus EPS (enteric coated)—by Jarrow

Acidophilus Pearls (enteric coated)—by Enzymatic Therapy

FiberSMART—by ReNew Life Formulas

Primadophilus Optima (enteric coated)—by Nature's Way

NSI Probiotic (enteric coated)—by Nutraceutical Sciences Institute/Vitacost

❧ Aloe Vera

Some Companies/Sources for This Plant Product

Lily of the Desert, Oasis, Platinum Health Products, Nature's Way

❧ Berry and Grape Extracts

Hawthorn Berry Solid Extract—by Gaia Herbs

Muscadine Grape Seed (pill)—by Nature's Pearl

MetaBerry—by Oasis

Goji 100 (berry juice)—by Genesis Today

Earth's Promise (powder, purple or elderberry)—by Enzymatic Therapy

Grape Seed Extracts

Grape Seed Phytosome—by Natural Factors

❧ Multivitamins, High Potency Pills (More Than Once a Day)

Opti-Packs, Super Blend, Perfect Blend, Women's Blend, Men's Blend—by Super Nutrition

Doctor's Choice series—by Enzymatic Therapy

MultiStart series (Dr. Michael Murray's formulas)—by Natural Factors

Advanced Nutritional System—by Rainbow Light

Complete Daily Pack—by Andrew Weil

❧ Multivitamins, Powders and Liquids

4 Total Nutrition (liquid)—by Genesis Today

Fatigued to Fantastic! Energy Revitalization System—by Enzymatic Therapy (powder, with B vitamins in a capsule; does not contain calcium)

❧ Multivitamins, Lower Potency Pills (Once a Day)

Men's One/Women's One/Menopause One/Active Senior—by Rainbow Light

Simply One Series—by Super Nutrition

Every Woman's One Daily—by New Chapter

Every Man's One Daily—by New Chapter

✍ Antioxidant Multiples

Ultimate Antioxidant—by Natural Factors
Antioxidants—by Pioneer
Antioxidant Power—by Super Nutrition
Anti-Oxidant Supreme—by Gaia Herbs
Select Formulas Antioxidant & Multivitamin—by Andrew Weil
Super 10 Antioxidant Formula—by Country Life

✍ Vitamin C

Ultra Gram C—by Rainbow Light
Vitamin C Complex—by Pioneer
Vitamin C—by Solaray

✍ Mixed Tocopherols

Vitamin E Full System Complete 8—by MegaFood
Super E+—by Pioneer
Natural Vitamin E—by Bluebonnet
Gamma E—by Source Naturals
Balanced E—by KAL

✍ Alpha-lipoic Acid

R-Lipoic Acid—by Source Naturals

Other Companies/Sources for This Supplement

Jarrow, Natural Factors, Solgar, Whole Foods

✆ Glucosamine

Glucosamine, Chondroitin, & MSM Complex—by Whole Foods (also contains bromelain and boswellin)

Glucosamine Chondroitin Joint Care Formula—by Pioneer (also contains MSM, gotu kola, bromelain, turmeric, and hawthorn)

Joint Vibrance—by Vibrant Health (glucosamine, chondroitin, MSM, collagen, grapeseed extract, curcumin, boswellin, etc.)

Glucosamine (alone)—by Enzymatic Therapy, Whole Foods

✆ MSM

Companies/Sources

Natural Factors, Whole Foods, Jarrow (powder)

✆ Enzymes—Digestive

Digest—by Enzymedica

Digest Gold (super strength)—by Enzymedica

Digestive Enzymes—by Pioneer

Multi Enzyme—by Natural Factors

Mega-Zyme (Original Formula), Mega-Zyme Dairy, Mega-Zyme Acid-Ease, etc.—by Enzymatic Therapy

Serrapeptase—by Physician Formulas

✆ Enzymes—Systemic (Proteolytic)

Repair (enteric coated)—by Enzymedica

Zymactive (enteric coated, Dr. Murray's formula)—by Natural Factors

Wobenzym (red tablet or clear tablet)—by Wobenzym

Serrapeptase—by Physician Formulas

✂ Bromelain

Super Bromelain (high potency)—by Bluebonnet
Bromelain—by Source Naturals

✂ Boswellia

Boswellia—by Solaray
Boswellia Extract—by Source Naturals

✂ Curcumin

Turmericforce—by New Chapter
Curcumin (or Itis-Care)—by Narula Research
Maximized Curcuminoids—by Vibrant Health
Curcumin 95—by Jarrow
Turmeric & Bromelain—by Natural Factors

✂ Gotu Kola

Gotu Kola (pills)—by Nature's Way
Gotu Kola Leaf & Root (liquid extract)—by Gaia Herbs

✂ Immune-Enhancing Multiples

Multiples to Consider When You're Coming Down with an Infection

TheraMend Recovery System—by Rainbow Light
Wellness Formula—by Source Naturals
System Well—by Nature's Way

Deep Health—by Herbs, Etc.
Host Defense—by New Chapter

❧ Growth Hormone Releasers/Pituitary Supporters

SomaLife gHP (pure, patented amino acid formula)—by SomaLife
GHS Max (patented amino acid formula)—by VesPro

Note: These are the only patented plant-derived HGH releasers on the market. The latter product also contains several botanicals, such as licorice and Southern bayberry.

❧ Mind-Supporting Supplements

Theanine

Crave-Relax (chewable theanine)—by Natural Factors
Sun Theanine—by Enzymatic Therapy

Ginkgo

Ginkgold—by Nature's Way
Ginkgo Bacopa Phytosome—by Natural Factors or Enzymatic Therapy
Ginkgo Extract—by Whole Foods

Formulas

Ginkgo-Bacopa Quick Thinking—by Rainbow Light
Bacopa-Ginkgo Brain Strength—by Planetary Formulas
Think Smart—by Whole Foods
Mental Alertness—by Gaia Herbs

Stress Formulas

B Complex Stress Formula—by Pioneer
Stress Support Multi—by New Chapter

Sleep Support

5-HTP (100 mg capsules)—by Source Naturals or Jarrow
Melatonin (time-release)—by Source Naturals
Deep Sleep (liquid herbal extract, capsule)—by Herbs, Etc.
Sound Sleep (liquid herbal extract, capsule)—by Gaia Herbs

Web sites for the above Companies/Sources

www.affordablesolaray.com (Solaray)
www.barleans.com (Barlean's)
www.carlsonlabs.com (Carlson Laboratories)
www.country-life.com (Country Life)
www.drweil.com (Dr. Weil's Web site)
www.enzy.com (Enzymatic Therapy)
www.enzymedica.com (Enzymedica)
www.gaiaherbs.com (Gaia Herbs)
www.genesistoday.net (Genesis Today)
www.greensplus.com (Greens+)
www.healthfromthesun.com (Health From The Sun)
www.herbsetc.com (Herbs, Etc.)
www.jarrow.com (Jarrow)
www.lilyofthedesert.com (Lily of the Desert)
www.megafood.com (MegaFood)
www.narularesearch.com (Narula Research)
www.naturalfactors.com (Natural Factors)
www.naturespearlproducts.com (Nature's Pearl)
www.naturesplus.com (Nature's Plus)
www.naturesway.com (Nature's Way)

www.newchapter.info (New Chapter)

www.nutraceutical.com (Solaray, KAL)

www.nordicnaturals.com (Nordic Naturals)

www.oasislifesciences.com (Oasis)

www.phporder.com/greens (Platinum Health Products)

www.physicianformulas.com (Physician Formulas)

www.pioneernutritional.com (Pioneer Nutritional Formulas)

www.planetaryformulas.com (Planetary Formulas)

www.renewlife.com (ReNew Life Formulas)

www.rainbowlight.com (Rainbow Light)

www.renewlife.com (Renew Life Formulas)

www.solgar.com (Solgar)

www.sourcenaturals.com (Source Naturals)

www.spectrumorganics.com (Spectrum Organic Products)

www.supernutritionusa.com (Super Nutrition)

www.thesecretsofyouth.com/pro/health/ (SomaLife)

www.trianglenutrition.com (Triangle Nutrition)

www.vespro.com/antiaging.php (VesPro)

www.viable-herbal.com (Viable Herbal Solutions)

www.vibranthealth.us (Vibrant Health)

www.vitacost.com (Nutraceutical Sciences Institute/Vitacost)

www.wholefoods.com (Whole Foods)

www.wobenzym.com (Wobenzym)

The above list is by no means intended to be the final word on supplements of value. Many health care professionals recommend and sell products from companies like Thorne and Metagenics, both of which are superb sources as well.

Appendix B
Integrative Medicine Resources

What follows is a list of reputable clinics, institutions, and organizations that can assist you in locating the best experts in integrative medicine.

American Holistic Health Association (AHHA)
The AHHA has compiled some extensive resource and referral lists to help locate holistic health care practitioners in your area and to assist you on your journey toward greater wellness. Click the "Resource & Referral Lists" section of the Web site.
Mailing address:
American Holistic Health Association
PO Box 17400
Anaheim, CA 92817-7400
Phone: (714) 779-6152
E-mail: mail@ahha.org
Web site: www.ahha.org

American Holistic Medical Association (AHMA)
The mission of the AHMA is to support health care practitioners in their evolving personal and professional development as healers and to educate physicians

about holistic medicine. The AHMA Web site provides an online database for locating holistic health practitioners.

Phone: (505) 292-7788

E-mail: info@holisticmedicine.org

Web site: www.holisticmedicine.org

American Osteopathic Association (AOA)

The AOA serves as the primary certifying body for osteopathic physicians (DOs) and is the accrediting agency for all osteopathic medical colleges and health care facilities. The Web site helps educate the public about the philosophy of osteopathic medicine and provides a link for locating DOs in your area.

Mailing address:

142 East Ontario Street

Chicago, IL 60611

Toll-free phone: (800) 621-1773

General phone: (312) 202-8000

Web site: www.osteopathic.org/index.cfm

Block Center for Integrative Cancer Care (BCICC)

Cancer presents unique challenges for postsurgery care. Directed by leading cancer specialist Keith I. Block, MD, this center offers a comprehensive clinical program for integrating the best of conventional treatments with therapeutic nutrition and other scientifically sound complementary therapies to enhance recovery and attain long-term survival. Because of its impressive track record, the Block center is widely regarded as the number one integrative cancer treatment facility in the U.S.

Mailing address:

Block Center for Integrative Cancer Care

1800 Sherman Avenue, Suite 515

Evanston, IL 60201

Phone: (847) 492-3040

Web site: www.blockmd.com

Columbia University's Integrative Medicine Program

This program, founded and directed by cardiothoracic surgeon and surgery professor Mehmet C. Oz, MD, is housed within Columbia's Department of Surgery and is helping to pave the way for the use of complementary therapies in the context of surgery. Dr. Oz's research interests include heart replacement surgery, minimally invasive cardiac surgery, and the use of complementary therapies to support cardiac patients attending Columbia's medical center.

Mailing address:

Integrative Medicine Program

Columbia University Medical Center

Milstein Hospital Building, 7-435

177 Fort Washington Avenue

New York, NY 10032

Phone: (212) 342-0002

Duke University's Center for Integrative Medicine

The center offers "individual patient consultation services, both public and professional education and dedicated research in the field of Integrative Medicine."

Mailing address:

Duke Center for Integrative Medicine

DUMC 3022

Durham, NC 27710

Phone: (919) 660-6826

Toll-free number: (866) 313-0959

George Washington University's Center for Integrative Medicine

The Center for Integrative Medicine at the GW Medical Center is dedicated to creating a healing environment in which patients have access to a variety of complementary and alternative therapies to promote healing and wellness. It also offers a "Prepare for Procedure/Surgery Program" that's firmly grounded in mind-body medicine.

Mailing address:

Center for Integrative Medicine

908 New Hampshire Ave Suite 200

Washington, DC 20037
Phone: (202) 833-5055
Web site: www.integrativemedicinedc.com/pl.html

Stress Reduction Program, Center for Mindfulness in Medicine, Health Care, and Society

This pioneering program, which is based at the University of Massachusetts, includes an in-depth stress reduction course that offers guided instruction in mindfulness meditation practices, mindful yoga practice, and inquiry exercises to enhance awareness in everyday life.

Mailing address:

Center for Mindfulness in Medicine, Health Care, and Society
University of Massachusetts Medical School
Shaw Building
55 Lake Avenue
Worcester North, MA 01655
E-mail: mindfulness@umassmed.edu
Phone: 508-856-2656
Web site: www.umassmed.edu/cfm/srp/

University of Arizona's Program in Integrative Medicine

The mission of this clinical and educational program, which was founded by Andrew Weil, MD, is "to lead the transformation of healthcare by creating, educating, and actively supporting a community of professionals who embody the philosophy and practice of Integrative Medicine."

Mailing address:

Program in Integrative Medicine
PO Box 245153
Tucson, AZ 85724-5153
Phone: (520) 626-6483
E-mail: piminfo@ahsc.arizona.edu
Web site: www.integrativemedicine.arizona.edu/

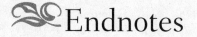

Endnotes

Chapter One: At the Cutting Edge of Surgical Care

1. Windsor A, Braga M, Martindale R, Buenos R, Tepaske R, Kraehenbuehl L, Weimann A. Fit for surgery: an expert panel review on optmising patients prior to surgery, with a particular focus on nutrition. Surgeon. 2004 Dec;2(6):315–9.

Chapter Two: The Art and Science of Wound Healing

1. Lee KA, Stotts, NA. Support of the growth hormone-somatomedin system to facilitate healing. Heart Lung. 1990;19(2):157–62.
2. Stadelmann WK, Digenis AG, Tobin GR. Impediments to wound healing. Am J Surg. 1998;176(2A Suppl):39S–47S.
3. Takano K, Mouri N, Sakurai H, Muto S, Koshizuka K, Tada Y. Effect of growth hormone on wound healing in protein-malnourished rats treated with corticosteroids. J Pediatr Surg. 1994 Jun;29(6):790–3.
4. Lioupis C. Effects of diabetes mellitus on wound healing: an update. J Wound Care. 2005 Feb;14(2):84–6.
5. Rai NK, Suryabhan, Ansari M, Kumar M, Shukla VK, Tripathi K. Effect of glycaemic control on apoptosis in diabetic wounds. J Wound Care. 2005 Jun;14(6):277–81; Bottermann P. Surgical operations in diabetics. MMW Fortschr Med. 2005 Sep 15;147(37):51–4.

6. Peppa M, Brem H, Ehrlich P, Zhang JG, Cai W, Li Z, Croitoru A, Thung S, Vlassara H. Adverse effects of dietary glycotoxins on wound healing in genetically diabetic mice. Diabetes. 2003 Nov;52(11):2805–13.

7. Adam K, Oswald I. Sleep helps healing. Br Med J (Clin Res Ed). 1984 Nov 24;289(6456):1400–1.

8. Evans JC, French DG. Sleep and healing in intensive care settings. Dimens Crit Care Nurs. 1995 Jul–Aug;14(4):189–99; North A. The effect of sleep on wound healing. Ostomy Wound Manage. 1990 Mar–Apr;27:56–8.

9. Harvey EJ, Agel J, Selznick HS, Chapman JR, Henley MB. Deleterious effect of smoking on healing of open tibia-shaft fractures. Am J Orthop. 2002;31(9):518–21; Ishikawa SN, Murphy GA, Richardson EG. The effect of cigarette smoking on hind-foot fusions. Foot Ankle Int. 2002;23(11):996–8; Mallon WJ, Misamore G, Snead DS, Denton P. The impact of preoperative smoking habits on the results of rotator cuff repair. J Shoulder Elbow Surg. 2004;13(2):129–32; Moller AM, Pedersen T, Villebro N, Munksgaard A. Effect of smoking on early complications after elective orthopedic surgery. J Bone Joint Surg Br. 2003; 85(2):178–81.

10. Sorensen LT, Horby J, Friis E, Pilsgaard B, Jorgensen T. Smoking as a risk factor for wound healing and infection in breast cancer surgery. Eur J Surg Oncol. 2002;28(8):815–20.

11. Manassa EH, Hertl CH, Olbrisch RR. Wound healing problems in smokers and non-smokers after 132 abdominoplasties. Plast Reconstr Surg. 2003 May;111(6):2082–7.

12. Akoz T, Akan M, Yildirim S. If you continue to smoke, we may have a problem: smoking's effects on plastic surgery. Aesthetic Plast Surg. 2002;26(6):477–82.

13. Warner MA et al. Preoperative cessation of smoking and pulmonary complications in coronoary artery bypass patients. Anesthisiology 1984; 60:380–3.

14. Whiteford L. Nicotine, CO and HCN: the detrimental effects of smoking on wound healing. Br J Community Nurs. 2003;8(12):S22–6.

15. Hornig DH, Glatthaar BE. Vitamin C and smoking: increased requirement of smokers. Int J Vitam Nutr Res Suppl. 1985;27:139–55.

16. Collins N. Adding vitamin C to the wound management mix. Adv Skin Wound Care. 2004;17(3):109–12.

17. Kiecolt-Glaser JK, Page GG, Marucha PT, MacCallum RC, Glaser R. Psychological influences on surgical recovery: perspectives from psychoneuroimmunology. Am Psychol. 1998;53(11):1209–18; Blankfield RP. Suggestion, relaxation, and hypnosis as adjuncts in the care of surgery patients: a review of the literature. Am J Clin Hypn. 1991;33(3):172–86.

18. Broadbent E, Petrie KJ, Alley PG, Booth RJ. Psychological stress impairs early wound repair following surgery. Psychosom Med. 2003;65(5):865–9.

19. Raholm MB. Weaving the fabric of spirituality as experienced by patients who have undergone a coronary bypass surgery. J Holist Nurs. 2002 Mar;20(1):31–47.

20. Boudreaux ED, O'Hea E, Chasuk R. Spiritual role in healing: an alternative way of

thinking. Prim Care. 2002 Jun;29(2):439–54; Lira LF. A clinical and spiritual approach to healing. Ostomy Wound Manage. 2004 Sep;50(9):15–6, 18; Harding OG. The healing power of intercessory prayer. West Indian Med J. 2001 Dec;50(4):269–72.

❧ Chapter Three: The Nutritional Foundation for Rapid Repair

1. Chopra, D. Creating Health: How to Wake Up the Body's Intelligence. Rev. ed. Boston: Mariner Books, 1995.

2. Eaton SB, Eaton SB 3rd, Konner MJ. Paleolithic nutrition revisited: a twelve-year retrospective on its nature and implications. Eur J Clin Nutr. 1997;51(4):207–16.

3. Eaton SB, Eaton SB 3rd. Paleolithic vs. modern diets—selected pathophysiological implications. Eur J Nutr. 2000;39(2):67–70.

4. King L. Impaired wound healing in patients with diabetes. Nurs Stand. 2001 Jun 6–12;15(38):39–45.

5. Ahmed N. Advanced glycation endproducts—role in pathology of diabetic complications. Diabetes Res Clin Pract. 2005 Jan;67(1):3–21.

6. Simopoulos AP. Evolutionary aspects of omega-3 fatty acids in the food supply. Prostaglandins Leukot Essent Fatty Acids. 1999;60(5–6):421–9.

7. Seaman DR. The diet-induced proinflammatory state: a cause of chronic pain and other degenerative diseases? J Manipulative Physiol Ther. 2002;25(3):168–79.

8. Collins N. Vegetarian diets and wound healing. Adv Skin Wound Care. 2003; 16(2):65–6.

9. Pawlosky RJ, Hibbeln JR, Novotny JA, Salem N Jr. Physiological compartmental analysis of alpha-linolenic acid metabolism in adult humans. J Lipid Res. 2001 Aug;42(8):1257–65.

10. Burdge GC, Wootton SA. Conversion of alpha-linolenic acid to eicosapentaenoic, docosapentaenoic and docosahexaenoic acids in young women. Br J Nutr. 2002; 88(4):411–20.

11. Davis BC, Kris-Etherton PM. Achieving optimal essential fatty acid status in vegetarians: current knowledge and practical implications. Am J Clin Nutr. 2003;78(3 Suppl):640S–646S.

12. Seaman DR. The diet-induced proinflammatory state: a cause of chronic pain and other degenerative diseases? J Manipulative Physiol Ther. 2002;25(3):168–79; Nutter RL. Gridley DS. Kettering JD. Andres ML. Aprecio RM. Slater JM. Modification of a transplantable colon tumor and immune responses in mice fed different sources of protein, fat and carbohydrate. Cancer Letters. 1983;18(1):49–62; Ludwig DS. Diet and development of the insulin resistance syndrome. Asia Pac J Clin Nutr. 2003;12 Suppl:S4.

13. Slavin J. Why whole grains are protective: biological mechanisms. Proc Nutr Soc. 2003 Feb;62(1):129–34.

14. Stephen AM. Whole grains—impact of consuming whole grains on physiological effects of dietary fiber and starch. Critical Reviews in Food Science & Nutrition. 1994;34(5–6):499–511.

15. Lang R, Jebb SA. Who consumes whole grains, and how much? Proc Nutr Soc. 2003 Feb;62(1):123–7.

16. Israelsen LD. Phytomedicines: the greening of modern medicine. Journal of Alternative & Complementary Medicine. 1995;1(3):245–8; Ren S. Lien EJ. Natural products and their derivatives as cancer chemopreventive agents. Progress in Drug Research. 1997;48:147–71.

17. Challem JJ. Toward a new definition of essential nutrients: is it now time for a third "vitamin" paradigm? Med Hypotheses. 1999 May;52(5):417–22.

18. Williamson EM. Synergy and other interactions in phytomedicines. Phytomedicine. 2001;8(5):401–9.

19. Fuhrman B, Volkova N, Rosenblat M, Aviram M. Lycopene synergistically inhibits LDL oxidation in combination with vitamin E, glabridin, rosmarinic acid, carnosic acid, or garlic. Antioxid Redox Signal. 2000;2(3):491–506.

20. Waladkhani AR, Clemens MR. Effect of dietary phytochemicals on cancer development (review). Int J Mol Med. 1998;1(4):747–53.

21. Calder PC. Long-chain n-3 fatty acids and inflammation: potential application in surgical and trauma patients. Braz J Med Biol Res. 2003 Apr;36(4):433–46; Sacks GS, Genton L, Kudsk KA. Controversy of immunonutrition for surgical critical-illness patients. Curr Opin Crit Care. 2003 Aug;9(4):300–5; Tsekos E, Reuter C, Stehle P, Boeden G. Perioperative administration of parenteral fish oil supplements in a routine clinical setting improves patient outcome after major abdominal surgery. Clin Nutr. 2004 Jun;23(3):325–30.

22. Heys SD, Ogston KN. Peri-operative nutritional support: controversies and debates. Int J Surg Investig. 2000;2(2):107–15.

23. MacBurney M, Young LS, Ziegler TR, Wilmore DW. A cost-evaluation of glutamine-supplemented parenteral nutrition in adult bone marrow transplant patients. J Am Diet Assoc. 1994;94(11):1263–6.

24. Brown SA, Goringe A, Fegan C, Davies SV, Giddings J, Whittaker JA, Burnett AK, Poynton CH. Parenteral glutamine protects hepatic function during bone marrow transplantation. Bone Marrow Transplant. 1998;22(3):281–4; Cockerham MB, Weinberger BB, Lerchie SB. Oral glutamine for the prevention of oral mucositis associated with high-dose paclitaxel and melphalan for autologous bone marrow transplantation. Ann Pharmacother. 2000;34(3):300–3.

25. Daly JM, Lieberman MD, Goldfine J, Shou J, Weintraub F, Rosato EF, Lavin P. Enteral nutrition with supplemental arginine, RNA, and omega-3 fatty acids in patients after operation: immunologic, metabolic, and clinical outcome. Surgery. 1992;112(1):56–67.

26. Bower RH, Cerra FB, Bershadsky B, Licari JJ, Hoyt DB, Jensen GL, Van Buren CT, Rothkopf MM, Daly JM, Adelsberg BR. Early enteral administration of a formula (Im-

pact) supplemented with arginine, nucleotides, and fish oil in intensive care unit patients: results of a multicenter, prospective, randomized, clinical trial. Crit Care Med. 1995;23(3):436–49; Daly JM, Lieberman MD, Goldfine J, Shou J, Weintraub F, Rosato EF, Lavin P. Enteral nutrition with supplemental arginine, RNA, and omega-3 fatty acids in patients after operation: immunologic, metabolic, and clinical outcome. Surgery. 1992;112(1):56–67; Gianotti L, Braga M, Vignali A, Balzano G, Zerbi A, Bisagni P, Di Carlo V. Effect of route of delivery and formulation of postoperative nutritional support in patients undergoing major operations for malignant neoplasms. Arch Surg. 1997 Nov;132(11):1222–9; Daly JM, Weintraub FN, Shou J, Rosato EF, Lucia M. Enteral nutrition during multimodality therapy in upper gastrointestinal cancer patients. Annals of Surgery. 1995;221(4):327–38.

27. Karmali RA. Historical perspective and potential use of n-3 fatty acids in therapy of cancer cachexia. Nutrition. 1996;12(1 Suppl):S2–4; Stehle P. Zander J. Mertes N. Albers S. Puchstein C. Lawin P. Furst P. Effect of parenteral glutamine peptide supplements on muscle glutamine loss and nitrogen balance after major surgery. Lancet. 1989;1(8632):231–3.

28. Nattakom TV, Charlton A, Wilmore DW. Use of vitamin E and glutamine in the successful treatment of severe veno-occlusive disease following bone marrow transplantation. Nutr Clin Pract. 1995;10(1):16–8.

✎ Chapter Four: Prepare to Repair

1. Astrup A, Meinert Larsen T, Harper A. Atkins and other low-carbohydrate diets: hoax or an effective tool for weight loss? Lancet. 2004 Sep 4;364(9437):897–9.

2. Godfrey RJ, Madgwick Z, Whyte GP. The exercise-induced growth hormone response in athletes. Sports Med. 2003;33(8):599–613.

3. Newsholme EA, Parry-Billings M. Properties of glutamine release from muscle and its importance for the immune system. JPEN J Parenter Enteral Nutr. 1990 Jul–Aug;14(4 Suppl):63S–67S; Parry-Billings M, Blomstrand E, McAndrew N, Newsholme EA. A communicational link between skeletal muscle, brain, and cells of the immune system. Int J Sports Med. 1990 May;11 Suppl 2:S122–8.

4. Calder PC. Long-chain n-3 fatty acids and inflammation: potential application in surgical and trauma patients. Braz J Med Biol Res. 2003 Apr;36(4):433–46.

5. Calder PC. Dietary modification of inflammation with lipids. Proc Nutr Soc. 2002 Aug;61(3):345–58.

6. Braga M, Gianotti L, Vignali A, Carlo VD. Preoperative oral arginine and n-3 fatty acid supplementation improves the immunometabolic host response and outcome after colorectal resection for cancer. Surgery. 2002 Nov;132(5):805–14.

7. Tsekos E, Reuter C, Stehle P, Boeden G. Perioperative administration of parenteral fish oil supplements in a routine clinical setting improves patient outcome after major abdominal surgery. Clin Nutr. 2004 Jun;23(3):325–30.

8. Marshall K. Therapeutic applications of whey protein. Altern Med Rev. 2004 Jun;9(2):136–156.

9. Zorrilla P, Salido JA, Lopez-Alonso A, Silva A. Serum zinc as a prognostic tool for wound healing in hip hemiarthroplasty. Clin Orthop. 2004 Mar;(420):304–8.

10. Elson ML. The role of retinoids in wound healing. J Am Acad Dermatol. 1998 Aug;39(2 pt. 3):S79–81.

11. Thomas DR. Specific nutritional factors in wound healing. Adv Wound Care. 1997 Jul–Aug; 10(4):40–3; Petry JJ. Surgically significant nutritional supplements. Plast Reconstr Surg. 1996 Jan;97(1):233–40.

12. Anstead GM. Steroids, retinoids, and wound healing. Adv Wound Care. 1998 Oct;11(6):277–85.

13. Talas DU, Nayci A, Atis S, Comelekoglu U, Polat A, Bagdatoglu C, Renda N. The effects of corticosteroids and vitamin A on the healing of tracheal anastomoses. Int J Pediatr Otorhinolaryngol. 2003 Feb;67(2):109–16.

14. Petry JJ. Surgically significant nutritional supplements. Plast Reconstr Surg. 1996;97(1):233–40.

15. Arend A, Zilmer M, Vihalemm T, Selstam G, Sepp E. Lipoic acid prevents suppression of connective tissue proliferation in the rat liver induced by n-3 PUFAs: a pilot study. Ann Nutr Metab. 2000;44(5-6):217–22.

16. Godfrey RJ, Madgwick Z, Whyte GP. The exercise-induced growth hormone response in athletes. Sports Med. 2003;33(8):599–613.

17. Broadbent E, Petrie KJ, Alley PG, Booth RJ. Psychological stress impairs early wound repair following surgery. Psychosom Med. 2003;65(5):865–9.

18. Kiecolt-Glaser JK, Page GG, Marucha PT, MacCallum RC, Glaser R. Psychological influences on surgical recovery. Perspectives from psychoneuroimmunology. Am Psychol. 1998;53(11):1209–18; Blankfield RP. Suggestion, relaxation, and hypnosis as adjuncts in the care of surgery patients: a review of the literature. Am J Clin Hypn. 1991;33(3):172–86.

19. White PF, Issioui T, Hu J, Jones SB, Coleman JE, Waddle JP, Markowitz SD, Coloma M, Macaluso AR, Ing CH. Comparative efficacy of acustimulation (ReliefBand) versus ondansetron (Zofran) in combination with droperidol for preventing nausea and vomiting. Anesthesiology. 2002 Nov;97(5):1075–81.

20. Coloma M, White PF, Ogunnaike BO, Markowitz SD, Brown PM, Lee AQ, Berrisford SB, Wakefield CA, Issioui T, Jones SB, Jones DB. Comparison of acustimulation and ondansetron for the treatment of established postoperative nausea and vomiting. Anesthesiology. 2002 Dec;97(6):1387–92.

21. Gan TJ, Jiao KR, Zenn M, Georgiade G. A randomized controlled comparison of electro-acupoint stimulation or ondansetron versus placebo for the prevention of postoperative nausea and vomiting. Anesth Analg. 2004 Oct;99(4):1070–5.

22. Kotani N, Hashimoto H, Sato Y, Sessler DI, Yoshioka H, Kitayama M, Yasuda T, Matsuki A. Preoperative intradermal acupuncture reduces postoperative pain, nausea and

vomiting, analgesic requirement, and sympathoadrenal responses. Anesthesiology. 2001 Aug;95(2):349–56.

❧ Chapter Five: Using Your Inner Healer During the Operation

1. Monte T. and editors of EastWest/Natural Health. Conventional modern medicine. In: World Medicine: The East West Guide to Healing Your Body. New York: Jeremy P. Tarcher/Perigree Books, 1993: p. 55.
2. Broadbent E, Petrie KJ, Alley PG, Booth RJ. Psychological stress impairs early wound repair following surgery. Psychosom Med. 2003;65(5):865–9.
3. Ibid.
4. Pert CB. The wisdom of the receptors: neuropeptides, the emotions, and bodymind. Adv Mind Body Med. 2002;18(1):30–5.
5. Benson H, Beary JF, Carol MP. The relaxation response. Psychiatry. 1974 Feb; 37(1):37–46.
6. Browner WS, Kahn AJ, Ziv E, Reiner AP, Oshima J, Cawthon RM, Hsueh WC, Cummings SR. The genetics of human longevity. Am J Med. 2004 Dec 1;117(11):851–60.
7. Broccoli D, Cooke H. Aging, healing, and the metabolism of telomeres. Am J Hum Genet. 1993 Apr;52(4):657–60.
8. Rudolph KL, Chang S, Lee HW, Blasco M, Gottlieb GJ, Greider C, DePinho RA. Longevity, stress response, and cancer in aging telomerase-deficient mice. Cell. 1999 Mar 5;96(5):701–12.
9. Aviv A. Telomeres and human aging: facts and fibs. Sci Aging Knowledge Environ. 2004 Dec 22;2004(51):pe43.
10. Epel ES, Blackburn EH, Lin J, Dhabhar FS, Adler NE, Morrow JD, Cawthon RM. Accelerated telomere shortening in response to life stress. Proc Natl Acad Sci USA. 2004 Dec 7;101(49):17312–5.
11. Esch T, Fricchione GL, Stefano GB. The therapeutic use of the relaxation response in stress-related diseases. Med Sci Monit. 2003 Feb;9(2):RA23–34; Kemeny ME, Gruenewald TL. Psychoneuroimmunology update. Semin Gastrointest Dis. 1999 Jan; 10(1):20–9.
12. Barrows KA, Jacobs BP. Mind-body medicine. An introduction and review of the literature. Med Clin North Am. 2002 Jan;86(1):11–31; Benson H, Greenwood MM, Klemchuk H. The relaxation response: psychophysiologic aspects and clinical applications. Int J Psychiatry Med. 1975; 6(1–2):87–98; Schaffer SD, Yucha CB. Relaxation and pain management: the relaxation response can play a role in managing chronic and acute pain. Am J Nurs. 2004 Aug;104(8):75–6, 78–9, 81–2.
13. Enqvist B, Fischer K. Preoperative hypnotic techniques reduce consumption of analgesics after surgical removal of third mandibular molars: a brief communication. Int J Clin Exp Hypn. 1997 Apr;45(2):102–8.

14. Shang AB, Gan TJ. Optimising postoperative pain management in the ambulatory patient. Drugs. 2003;63(9):855–67; Barrows KA, Jacobs BP. Med Clin North Am. 2002; 86(1):11–31; op cit.

15. Rapkin DA, Straubing M, Holroyd JC. Guided imagery, hypnosis and recovery from head and neck cancer surgery: an exploratory study. Int J Clin Exp Hypn. 1991 Oct;39(4):215–26; Pinnell CM, Covino NA. Empirical findings on the use of hypnosis in medicine: a critical review. Int J Clin Exp Hypn. 2000 Apr;48(2):170–94; Lynn SJ, Kirsch I, Barabasz A, Cardena E, Patterson D. Hypnosis as an empirically supported clinical intervention: the state of the evidence and a look to the future. Int J Clin Exp Hypn. 2000 Apr;48(2):239–59; Blankfield RP. Suggestion, relaxation, and hypnosis as adjuncts in the care of surgery patients: a review of the literature. Am J Clin Hypn. 1991 Jan;33(3):172–86.

16. Ginandes C, Brooks P, Sando W, Jones C, Aker J. Can medical hypnosis accelerate post-surgical wound healing? Results of a clinical trial. Am J Clin Hypn. 2003 Apr;45(4):333–51.

17. Meurisse M, Defechereux T, Hamoir E, Maweja S, Marchettini P, Gollogly L, Degauque C, Joris J, Faymonville ME. Hypnosis with conscious sedation instead of general anaesthesia? Applications in cervical endocrine surgery. Acta Chir Belg. 1999 Aug;99(4):151–8.

18. Holden-Lund C. Effects of relaxation with guided imagery on surgical stress and wound healing. Res Nurs Health. 1988 Aug;11(4):235–44.

19. Evans C, Richardson PH. Improved recovery and reduced postoperative stay after - therapeutic suggestions during general anaesthesia. Lancet. 1988 Aug 27;2(8609): 491–3.

20. Ginandes CS, Rosenthal DI. Related Using hypnosis to accelerate the healing of bone fractures: a randomized controlled pilot study. Altern Ther Health Med. 1999 Mar;5(2): 67–75; Ginandes C, Brooks P, Sando W, Jones C, Aker J. Can medical hypnosis accelerate post-surgical wound healing? Results of a clinical trial.Am J Clin Hypn. 2003 Apr;45(4): 333–51.

21. Ginandes CS. The strategic integration of hypnosis and CBT for the treatment of mind/body conditions. In: Chapman R (ed.). The Clinical Use of Hypnosis in Cognitive Behavior Therapy: A Practitioners Casebook. New York: Springer Publications, 2005.

22. Ginandes C. Rapid Recovery from Injury. CD audio. Akron, Ohio: Health Journeys (Web site: www.healthjourneys.com), 2005; Ginandes C. Preparation and Recovery from Surgery. 2 CD audio program. E-mail: cginandes@aol.com; Phone: 617–924–4093. 2005.

23. De Paula AA, de Carvalho EC, dos Santos CB. The use of the "progressive muscle relaxation" technique for pain relief in gynecology and obstetrics. Rev Lat Am Enfermagem. 2002 Sep–Oct;10(5): 654–9.

24. Mandle CL, Domar AD, Harrington DP, Leserman J, Bozadjian EM, Friedman R,

Benson H. Relaxation response in femoral angiography. Radiology. 1990 Mar;174(3 pt. 1): 737–9.

25. Mandle CL, Jacobs SC, Arcari PM, Domar AD. The efficacy of relaxation response interventions with adult patients: a review of the literature. J Cardiovasc Nurs. 1996 Apr;10(3): 4–26.

26. Hudesman J, Tjeuw M, Collins P. Responsiveness to verbal instruction during anesthesia: a pilot report. Percept Mot Skills. 1991 Apr;72(2): 424–6.

27. Block RI, Ghoneim MM, Sum Ping ST, Ali MA. Human learning during general anaesthesia and surgery. Br J Anaesth. 1991 Feb;66(2): 170–8.

28. Schwender D, Klasing S, Faber-Zullig E, Poppel E, Peter K. Conscious and unconscious acoustic perception during general anesthesia. Anaesthesist. 1991 Nov;40(11): 583–93.

29. McLintock TT, Aitken H, Downie CF, Kenny GN. Postoperative analgesic requirements in patients exposed to positive intraoperative suggestions. BMJ. 1990 Oct 6;301(6755): 788–90.

30. Evans C, Richardson PH. Improved recovery and reduced postoperative stay after therapeutic suggestions during general anaesthesia. Lancet. 1988 Aug 27;2(8609): 491–3.

31. Steinberg ME, Hord AH, Reed B, Sebels PS. Study of the effect of intraoperative analgesia and wellbeing. In: Memory and Awareness in Anesthesia. Englewood Cliffs, NJ: Prentice Hall, 1993.

32. Lebovits AH, Twersky R, McEwan B. Intraoperative therapeutic suggestions in daycase surgery: are there benefits for postoperative outcome? Br J Anaesth. 1999 Jun;82(6): 861–6.

33. Fife D, Rappaport E. Noise and hospital stay. Am J Public Health. 1976 Jul;66(7): 680–1.

34. Wang SM, Kulkarni L, Dolev J, Kain ZN. Music and preoperative anxiety: a randomized, controlled study. Anesth Analg. 2002 Jun;94(6): 1489–94; Cooke M, Chaboyer W, Hiratos MA. Music and its effect on anxiety in short waiting periods: a critical appraisal. J Clin Nurs. 2005 Feb;14(2): 145–55; Chan YM, Lee PW, Ng TY, Ngan HY, Wong LC. The use of music to reduce anxiety for patients undergoing colposcopy: a randomized trial. Gynecol Oncol. 2003 Oct;91(1): 213–7; Nilsson U, Rawal N, Enqvist B, Unosson M. Analgesia following music and therapeutic suggestions in the PACU in ambulatory surgery; a randomized controlled trial. Acta Anaesthesiol Scand. 2003 Mar;47(3): 278–83.

35. Voss JA, Good M, Yates B, Baun MM, Thompson A, Hertzog M. Sedative music reduces anxiety and pain during chair rest after open-heart surgery. Pain. 2004 Nov;112(1–2): 197–203.

36. Nilsson U, Rawal N, Unestahl LE, Zetterberg C, Unosson M. Improved recovery after music and therapeutic suggestions during general anaesthesia: a double-blind randomised controlled trial. Acta Anaesthesiol Scand. 2001 Aug;45(7): 812–7.

37. Phillips SJ. Physiology of wound healing and surgical wound care. ASAIO J. 2000; 46(6): S2–5.

38. Crowley LV, Seifter E, Kriss P, Rettura G, Nakao K, Levenson SM. Effects of enviromental temperature and femoral fracture on wound healing in rats. J Trauma. 1977 Jun;17(6): 436–45.

39. Leslie K, Sessler DI. Perioperative hypothermia in the high-risk surgical patient. Best Pract Res Clin Anaesthesiol. 2003 Dec;17(4): 485–98.

40. Kurz A, Sessler DI, Lenhardt R. Perioperative normothermia to reduce the incidence of surgical-wound infection and shorten hospitalization. Engl J Med. 1996 May 9;334(19): 1209–15.

41. Schilling J. Wound healing. Surg Round 1983;6: 46–62.

42. Whitney JD. Supplemental perioperative oxygen and fluids to improve surgical wound outcomes: translating evidence into practice. Wound Repair Regen 2003; 11(6): 462–7.

43. Tandara AA, Mustoe TA. Oxygen in wound healing—more than a nutrient. World J Surg. 2004; 28(3):294–300.

44. Lombardi AV Jr., Berend KR, Mallory TH. Perioperative Management—Rapid Recovery Protocol. In: Breusch SJ, Malchau H (ed.). The Well Cemented Total Hip Arthroplasty—Theory and Practice, chap. 13, pp. 307–312. Heidelberg, Germany: Springer Verlag, 2005.

45. Berend KR, Lombardi AV Jr, Mallory TH. Rapid recovery protocol for peri-operative care of total hip and total knee arthroplasty patients. Surg Technol Int. 2004;13:239–47.

46. Goodman S. Therapeutic effects of organic germanium. Med Hypotheses. 1988 Jul;26(3):207–15.

47. Broussard CL. Hyperbaric oxygenation and wound healing. J Vasc Nurs. 2004; 22(2):42–8.

48. Yildiz S, Uluutku H, Gunay A, Yildirim I, Yildirim S, Gurbuz AK. The effect of hyperbaric oxygen therapy on the adverse effects of octreotide on wound healing. Eur J Gastroenterol Hepatol. 2004 May;16(5):475–8.

49. Kranke P, Bennett M, Roeckl-Wiedmann I, Debus S. Hyperbaric oxygen therapy for chronic wounds. Cochrane Database Syst Rev. 2004;(2):CD004123.

50. Cianci P. Advances in the treatment of the diabetic foot: is there a role for adjunctive hyperbaric oxygen therapy? Wound Repair Regen. 2004 Jan–Feb;12(1):2–10; Kessler L, Bilbault P, Ortega F, Grasso C, Passemard R, Stephan D, Pinget M, Schneider F. Hyperbaric oxygenation accelerates the healing rate of nonischemic chronic diabetic foot ulcers: a prospective randomized study. Diabetes Care. 2003; 26(8):2378–82.

51. Gottrup F. Oxygen in wound healing and infection. World J Surg. 2004; 28(3):312–5.

52. Knaster M. Discovering the Body's Wisdom. New York: Bantam, 1996.

53. Papantonio C. Alternative medicine and wound healing. Ostomy Wound Manage. 1998 Apr;44(4):44–6, 48, 50; Wirth DP, Richardson JT, Eidelman WS. Wound heal-

ing and complementary therapies: a review. J Altern Complement Med. 1996 Winter;2(4):493–502.

54. Palmer RF, Katerndahl D, Morgan-Kidd J. A randomized trial of the effects of remote intercessory prayer: interactions with personal beliefs on problem-specific outcomes and functional status. J Altern Complement Med. 2004 Jun;10(3):438–48.

55. Lira LF. A clinical and spiritual approach to healing. Ostomy Wound Manage. 2004 Sep;50(9):15–6, 18.

⁇ Chapter Six: Preventing Postoperative Complications

1. Anand KJ. The stress response to surgical trauma: from physiological basis to therapeutic implications. Prog Food Nutr Sci. 1986;10(1–2):67–132.

2. Ibid.

3. Anonymous. Muscle provides glutamine to the immune system. Nutr Rev. 1990 Oct;48(10):390–2; Newsholme EA, Parry-Billings M. Properties of glutamine release from muscle and its importance for the immune system. JPEN J Parenter Enteral Nutr. 1990 Jul–Aug;14(4 Suppl):63S–67S.

4. Nicholson G, Hall GM, Burrin JM. Peri-operative steroid supplementation. Anaesthesia 1998;53(11):1091–1104.

5. Han JS. Acupuncture and endorphins. Neurosci Lett. 2004 May 6;361(1–3):258–61; Cao X. Scientific bases of acupuncture analgesia. Acupunct Electrother Res. 2002;27(1):1–14; Domangue BB, Margolis CG, Lieberman D, Kaji H. Biochemical correlates of hypnoanalgesia in arthritic pain patients. J Clin Psychiatry. 1985 Jun;46(6):235–8.

6. Kaada B, Torsteinbo O. Increase of plasma beta-endorphins in connective tissue massage. Gen Pharmacol. 1989;20(4):487–9.

7. Kehlet H. Multimodal approach to control postoperative pathophysiology and rehabilitation. Br J Anaesth. 1997;78:606–17.

8. Mangano DT, Hollenberg M, Fegert G, et al. Perioperative myocardial ischemia in patients undergoing noncardiac surgery—I: Incidence and severity during the 4-day perioperative period. The Study of Perioperative Ischemia (SPI) Research Group. J Am Coll Cardiol. 1991;17:843–850.

9. Fugh-Berman A. Herbs and dietary supplements in the prevention and treatment of cardiovascular disease. Prev Cardiol. 2000 Winter;3(1):24–32.

10. Fong HH, Bauman JL. Hawthorn. J Cardiovasc Nurs. 2002 Jul;16(4):1–8; Rigelsky JM, Sweet BV. Hawthorn: pharmacology and therapeutic uses. Am J Health Syst Pharm. 2002 Mar 1;59(5):417–22.

11. Kearon C. Perioperative management of long-term anticoagulation. Seminars in Thrombosis and Hemostasis. 1998; 24 Suppl 1:77–83.

12. Dunn AS, Turpie AG. Perioperative management of patients receiving oral anticoagulants: a systematic review. Arch Intern Med. 2003 Apr 28;163(8):901–8.

13. Otley CC. Continuation of medically necessary aspirin and warfarin during cutaneous surgery. Mayo Clin Proc. 2003 Nov;78(11):1392–6.

14. Cobas M. Preoperative assessment of coagulation disorders. International Anesthesiology Clinics. 2001; 39(1):1–15.

15. Jiang X, Williams KM, Liauw WS, Ammit AJ, Roufogalis BD, Duke CC, Day RO, McLachlan AJ. Effect of ginkgo and ginger on the pharmacokinetics and pharmacodynamics of warfarin in healthy subjects. Br J Clin Pharmacol. 2005 Apr;59(4):425–32.

16. Yuan CS, Wei G, Dey L, Karrison T, Nahlik L, Maleckar S, Kasza K, Ang-Lee M, Moss J. Brief communication: American ginseng reduces warfarin's effect in healthy patients: a randomized, controlled Trial. Ann Intern Med. 2004;141(1):23–7.

17. Lee A, Done ML. Stimulation of the wrist acupuncture point P6 for preventing postoperative nausea and vomiting. Cochrane Database Syst Rev. 2004;(3):CD003281.

18. Kim Y, Kim CW, Kim KS. Clinical observations on postoperative vomiting treated by auricular acupuncture. Am J Chin Med. 2003;31(3):475–80.

19. Schneider A, Lowe B, Streitberger K. Perception of bodily sensation as a predictor of treatment response to acupuncture for postoperative nausea and vomiting prophylaxis. J Altern Complement Med. 2005 Feb;11(1):119–25.

20. Schlager A, Offer T, Baldissera I. Laser stimulation of acupuncture point P6 reduces postoperative vomiting in children undergoing strabismus surgery. Br J Anaesth. 1998 Oct;81(4):529–32.

21. Rusy LM, Hoffman GM, Weisman SJ. Electroacupuncture prophylaxis of postoperative nausea and vomiting following pediatric tonsillectomy with or without adenoidectomy. Anesthesiology. 2002 Feb;96(2):300–5.

22. Butkovic D, Toljan S, Matolic M, Kralik S, Radesic L. Comparison of laser acupuncture and metoclopramide in PONV prevention in children. Paediatr Anaesth. 2005 Jan;15(1):37–40.

23. Alkaissi A, Evertsson K, Johnsson VA, Ofenbartl L, Kalman S. P6 acupressure may relieve nausea and vomiting after gynecological surgery: an effectiveness study in 410 women. Can J Anaesth. 2002 Dec;49(10):1034–9; Alkaissi A, Stalnert M, Kalman S. Effect and placebo effect of acupressure (P6) on nausea and vomiting after outpatient gynaecological surgery. Acta Anaesthesiol Scand. 1999 Mar;43(3):270–4; Boehler M, Mitterschiffthaler G, Schlager A. Korean hand acupressure reduces postoperative nausea and vomiting after gynecological laparoscopic surgery. Anesth Analg. 2002 Apr;94(4):872–5.

24. Schlager A, Boehler M, Puhringer F. Korean hand acupressure reduces postoperative vomiting in children after strabismus surgery. Br J Anaesth. 2000 Aug;85(2):267–70.

25. Chen LL, Hsu SF, Wang MH, Chen CL, Lin YD, Lai JS. Use of acupressure to improve gastrointestinal motility in women after trans-abdominal hysterectomy. Am J Chin Med. 2003;31(5):781–90.

26. Koretz RL, Rotblatt M. Complementary and alternative medicine in gastroenterology: the good, the bad, and the ugly. Clin Gastroenterol Hepatol. 2004 Nov;2(11):957–67.

27. Lee A, Done ML. The use of nonpharmacologic techniques to prevent postoperative nausea and vomiting: a meta-analysis. Anesth Analg. 1999 Jun;88(6):1362–9.

28. Enqvist B, Bjorklund C, Engman M, Jakobsson J. Preoperative hypnosis reduces post-operative vomiting after surgery of the breasts: a prospective, randomized and blinded study. Acta Anaesthesiol Scand. 1997 Sep;41(8):1028–32.

29. Liu S, Carpenter RL, Neal JM. Epidural anesthesia and analgesia. Their role in post-operative outcome. Anesthesiology 1995; 82:1474–1506.

30. Moller JT, Cluitmans P, Rasmussen LS, et al, for the ISPOCD investigators. Long-term postoperative cognitive dysfunction in the elderly ISPOCD1 study. International Study of Post-Operative Cognitive Dysfunction. Lancet. 1998;351:857–61.

31. Rohan D, Buggy DJ, Crowley S, Ling FK, Gallagher H, Regan C, Moriarty DC. Increased incidence of postoperative cognitive dysfunction 24 hr after minor surgery in the elderly. Can J Anaesth. 2005 Feb;52(2):137–42.

32. Raja PV, Blumenthal JA, Doraiswamy PM. Cognitive deficits following coronary artery bypass grafting: prevalence, prognosis, and therapeutic strategies. CNS Spectr. 2004 Oct;9(10):763–72.

33. Kadoi Y, Saito S, Fujita N, Goto F. Risk factors for cognitive dysfunction after coronary artery bypass graft surgery in patients with type 2 diabetes. J Thorac Cardiovasc Surg. 2005 Mar;129(3):576–83.

34. Muller SV, Krause N, Schmidt M, Munte TF, Munte S. Cognitive dysfunction after abdominal surgery in elderly patients. Z Gerontol Geriatr. 2004 Dec;37(6):475–85.

35. Rohan D, Buggy DJ, Crowley S, Ling FK, Gallagher H, Regan C, Moriarty DC. Increased incidence of postoperative cognitive dysfunction 24 hr after minor surgery in the elderly. Can J Anaesth. 2005 Feb;52(2):137–42.

36. Wu CL, Hsu W, Richman JM, Raja SN. Postoperative cognitive function as an outcome of regional anesthesia and analgesia. Reg Anesth Pain Med. 2004 May–Jun;29(3):257–68.

37. Gertz HJ, Kiefer M. Review about Ginkgo biloba special extract EGb 761 (Ginkgo). Curr Pharm Des. 2004;10(3):261–4; Yoshikawa T, Naito Y, Kondo M. Ginkgo biloba leaf extract: review of biological actions and clinical applications. Antioxid Redox Signal. 1999 Winter;1(4):469–80; Birks J, Grimley EV, Van Dongen M. Ginkgo biloba for cognitive impairment and dementia. Cochrane Database Syst Rev. 2002;(4):CD003120.

38. Mix JA, Crews WD Jr. An examination of the efficacy of Ginkgo biloba extract EGb761 on the neuropsychologic functioning of cognitively intact older adults. J Altern Complement Med. 2000 Jun;6(3):219–29; Rigney U, Kimber S, Hindmarch I. The effects of acute doses of standardized Ginkgo biloba extract on memory and psychomotor performance in volunteers. Phytother Res. 1999 Aug;13(5):408–15; Mix JA, Crews WD Jr. A double-blind, placebo-controlled, randomized trial of Ginkgo biloba

extract EGb 761 in a sample of cognitively intact older adults: neuropsychological findings. Hum Psychopharmacol. 2002 Aug;17(6):267–77.

39. Kidd PM. A review of nutrients and botanicals in the integrative management of cognitive dysfunction. Altern Med Rev. 1999 Jun;4(3):144–61.

40. Pepeu G, Spignoli G. Nootropic drugs and brain cholinergic mechanisms. Prog Neuropsychopharmacol Biol Psychiatry. 1989;13 Suppl:S77–88.

41. Maggioni M, Picotti GB, Bondiolotti GP, Panerai A, Cenacchi T, Nobile P, Brambilla F. Effects of phosphatidylserine therapy in geriatric patients with depressive disorders. Acta Psychiatr Scand. 1990 Mar;81(3):265–70.

42. Pepeu G, Pepeu IM, Amaducci L. A review of phosphatidylserine pharmacological and clinical effects. Is phosphatidylserine a drug for the ageing brain? Pharmacol Res. 1996 Feb;33(2):73–80; Crook TH, Tinklenberg J, Yesavage J, Petrie W, Nunzi MG, Massari DC. Effects of phosphatidylserine in age-associated memory impairment. Neurology. 1991 May;41(5):644–9.

43. Moriguchi T, Greiner RS, Salem N Jr. Behavioral deficits associated with dietary induction of decreased brain docosahexaenoic acid concentration. J Neurochem. 2000 Dec;75(6): 2563–73.

44. Kalmijn S, van Boxtel MP, Ocke M, Verschuren WM, Kromhout D, Launer LJ. Dietary intake of fatty acids and fish in relation to cognitive performance at middle age. Neurology. 2004 Jan 27;62(2):275–80.

45. Bourre JM. Dietary Omega-3 Fatty Acids and Psychiatry: Mood, Behaviour, Stress, Depression, Dementia and Aging. J Nutr Health Aging. 2005;9(1):31–38; Casper RC. Nutrients, neurodevelopment, and mood. Curr Psychiatry Rep. 2004 Dec;6(6):425–9.

46. Belayev L, Marcheselli VL, Khoutorova L, Rodriguez de Turco EB, Busto R, Ginsberg MD, Bazan NG. Docosahexaenoic acid complexed to albumin elicits high-grade ischemic neuroprotection. Stroke. 2005 Jan;36(1):118–23.

47. Morris J, Royle GT. Choice of surgery for early breast cancer: pre- and postoperative levels of clinical anxiety and depression in patients and their husbands. Br J Surg. 1987 Nov;74(11):1017–9; Blacher RS. "It isn't fair": postoperative depression and other manifestations of survivor guilt. Gen Hosp Psychiatry. 2000 Jan–Feb;22(1): 43–8.

48. Rothenhausler HB, Grieser B, Nollert G, Reichart B, Schelling G, Kapfhammer HP. Psychiatric and psychosocial outcome of cardiac surgery with cardiopulmonary bypass: a prospective 12-month follow-up study. Gen Hosp Psychiatry. 2005 Jan–Feb;27(1):18–28.

49. Szekely A, Benko E, Varga A, Meszaros R. Postoperative depression after open heart surgery. Orv Hetil. 2001 Oct 14;142(41):2263–5.

50. Voulgari A, Papanikolaou MN, Lykouras L, Alevizos B, Alexiou E, Christodoulou GN. Prevention of postoperative anxiety and depression. Bibl Psychiatr. 1994;(165):49–55.

51. Bottiglieri T, Hyland K, Reynolds EH. The clinical potential of ademetionine (S-adenosylmethionine) in neurological disorders. Drugs. 1994 Aug;48(2):137–52;

Fugh-Berman A, Cott JM. Dietary supplements and natural products as psychotherapeutic agents. Psychosom Med. 1999 Sep–Oct;61(5):712–28.

52. Stough C, Lloyd J, Clarke J, Downey LA, Hutchison CW, Rodgers T, Nathan PJ. The chronic effects of an extract of Bacopa monniera (Brahmi) on cognitive function in healthy human subjects. Psychopharmacology (Berl). 2001 Aug;156(4):481–4; Vohora D, Pal SN, Pillai KK Protection from phenytoin-induced cognitive deficit by Bacopa monniera, a reputed Indian nootropic plant. J Ethnopharmacol. 2000 Aug;71(3):383–90; Roodenrys S, Booth D, Bulzomi S, Phipps A, Micallef C, Smoker J. Chronic effects of Brahmi (Bacopa monnieri) on human memory. Neuropsychopharmacology. 2002 Aug; 27(2):279–81.

53. Larzelere MM, Wiseman P. Anxiety, depression, and insomnia. Prim Care. 2002 Jun;29(2):339–60.

54. Birdsall TC. 5-Hydroxytryptophan: a clinically-effective serotonin precursor. Altern Med Rev. 1998 Aug;3(4):271–80.

55. Sprinkle PM, McClung JE, Paine JA. The immunocompromised human host: diagnosis and treatment. Laryngoscope. 1985 Apr;95(4):397–400; McIrvine AJ, Mannick JA. Lymphocyte function in the critically ill surgical patient. Surg Clin North Am. 1983 Apr;63(2):245–61.

56. Dauch WA, Krex D, Heymanns J, Zeithammer B, Bauer BL. Peri-operative changes of cellular and humoral components of immunity with brain tumour surgery. Acta Neurochir (Wien). 1994;126(2–4):93–101; Cheadle WG, Mercer-Jones M, Heinzelmann M, Polk HC Jr. Sepsis and septic complications in the surgical patient: who is at risk? Shock. 1996;6 Suppl 1:S6–9.

57. Penn I. Depressed immunity and the development of cancer. Cancer Detect Prev. 1994;18(4):241–52.

58. Heidecke CD, Weighardt H, Hensler T, Bartels H, Holzmann B. Immune paralysis of T-lymphocytes and monocytes in postoperative abdominal sepsis. Correlation of immune function with survival. Chirurg. 2000 Feb;71(2):159–65.

59. Hall JC, Heel K, McCauley R. Glutamine. Br J Surg. 1996 Mar;83(3):305–12.

60. Griffiths RD. The evidence for glutamine use in the critically-ill. Proc Nutr Soc. 2001 Aug;60(3):403–10.

61. Wilmore DW. The effect of glutamine supplementation in patients following elective surgery and accidental injury. J Nutr. 2001 Sep;131(9 Suppl):2543S–9S.

62. Newsholme P. Why is L-glutamine metabolism important to cells of the immune system in health, postinjury, surgery or infection? J Nutr. 2001 Sep;131(9 Suppl): 2515S–22S.

63. Quan ZF, Yang C, Li N, Li JS. Effect of glutamine on change in early postoperative intestinal permeability and its relation to systemic inflammatory response. World J Gastroenterol. 2004 Jul 1;10(13):1992–4; Wilmore DW, Smith RJ, O'Dwyer ST, Jacobs DO, Ziegler TR, Wang XD. The gut: a central organ after surgical stress. Surgery. 1988 Nov;104(5):917–23.

64. O'Flaherty L, Bouchier-Hayes DJ. Immunonutrition and surgical practice. Proc Nutr Soc. 1999 Nov;58(4):831–7; Sacks GS, Genton L, Kudsk KA. Controversy of immunonutrition for surgical critical-illness patients. Curr Opin Crit Care. 2003 Aug;9(4):300–5; Heyland DK, Novak F, Drover JW, Jain M, Su X, Suchner U. Should immunonutrition become routine in critically ill patients? A systematic review of the evidence. JAMA. 2001 Aug 22–29;286(8):944–53; Grimble RF. Immunonutrition. Curr Opin Gastroenterol. 2005 Mar;21(2):216–22.

65. Montejo JC, Zarazaga A, Lopez-Martinez J, Urrutia G, Roque M, Blesa AL, Celaya S, Conejero R, Galban C, Garcia de Lorenzo A, Grau T, Mesejo A, Ortiz-Leyba C, Planas M, Ordonez J, Jimenez FJ; Spanish Society of Intensive Care Medicine and Coronary Units. Immunonutrition in the intensive care unit. A systematic review and consensus statement. Clin Nutr. 2003 Jun;22(3):221–33.

66. Apfelbaum JL, Chen C, Mehta SS, Gan TJ. Postoperative pain experience: results from a national survey suggest postoperative pain continues to be undermanaged. Anesth Analg. 2003;97:534–540.

67. Kehlet H. Multimodal approach to control postoperative pathophysiology and rehabilitation. Br J Anaesth. 1997;78:606–17.

68. Jorgensen H, Wetterslev J, Moiniche S, Dahl JB. Epidural local anaesthetics versus opioid-based analgesic regimens on postoperative gastrointestinal paralysis, PONV and pain after abdominal surgery. Cochrane Database Syst Rev. 2000;(4):CD001893.

69. Hahnenkamp K, Herroeder S, Hollmann MW. Regional anaesthesia, local anaesthetics and the surgical stress response. Best Pract Res Clin Anaesthesiol. 2004 Sep;18(3):509–27; Grass JA. The role of epidural anesthesia and analgesia in postoperative outcome. Anesthesiol Clin North America. 2000 Jun;18(2):407–28.

70. Chumbley GM, Ward L, Hall GM, Salmon P. Pre-operative information and patient-controlled analgesia: much ado about nothing. Anaesthesia. 2004 Apr;59(4):354–8.

71. Vallejo R, de Leon-Casasola O, Benyamin R. Opioid therapy and immunosuppression: a review. Am J Ther. 2004 Sep–Oct;11(5):354–65.

72. Murray JB. Evidence for acupuncture's analgesic effectiveness and proposals for the physiological mechanisms involved. J Psychol. 1995 Jul;129(4):443–61.

73. Lin JG, Lo MW, Wen YR, Hsieh CL, Tsai SK, Sun WZ. The effect of high and low frequency electroacupuncture in pain after lower abdominal surgery. Pain. 2002 Oct;99(3):509–14; Sim CK, Xu PC, Pua HL, Zhang G, Lee TL. Effects of electroacupuncture on intraoperative and postoperative analgesic requirement. Acupunct Med. 2002 Aug;20(2–3):56–65; Wang B, Tang J, White PF, Naruse R, Sloninsky A, Kariger R, Gold J, Wender RH. Effect of the intensity of transcutaneous acupoint electrical stimulation on the postoperative analgesic requirement. Anesth Analg. 1997 Aug;85(2):406–13.

74. Kotani N, Hashimoto H, Sato Y, Sessler DI, Yoshioka H, Kitayama M, Yasuda T, Matsuki A. Preoperative intradermal acupuncture reduces postoperative pain, nausea and

vomiting, analgesic requirement, and sympathoadrenal responses. Anesthesiology. 2001 Aug;95(2):349–56.

75. Kaptchuk TJ. Acupuncture: theory, efficacy, and practice. Ann Intern Med. 2002 Mar 5;136(5):374–83.

76. Chen L, Tang J, White PF, Sloninsky A, Wender RH, Naruse R, Kariger R. The effect of location of transcutaneous electrical nerve stimulation on postoperative opioid analgesic requirement: acupoint versus nonacupoint stimulation. Anesth Analg. 1998 Nov;87(5):1129–34.

77. Rakel B, Frantz R. Effectiveness of transcutaneous electrical nerve stimulation on postoperative pain with movement. J Pain. 2003 Oct;4(8):455–64.

78. Redmond M, Florence B, Glass PS. Effective analgesic modalities for ambulatory patients. Anesthesiol Clin North America. 2003 Jun;21(2):329–46; Nissel H. Pain treatment by means of acupuncture. Acupunct Electrother Res. 1993 Jan–Mar;18(1):1–8.

79. Shang AB, Gan TJ. Optimising postoperative pain management in the ambulatory patient. Drugs. 2003;63(9):855–67

❧ Chapter Seven: Rapid Repair for the Postoperative Period

1. Edwards SL. Malnutrition in hospital patients: where does it come from? Br J Nurs. 1998 Sep 10–23;7(16):954–8, 971–4; Holmes S. Undernutrition in hospital patients. Nurs Stand. 2003;17(19):45–52.

2. Aznarte Padial P, Pareja Rodriguez de Vera A, de la Rubia Nieto A, Lopez Soriano F, Martinez de Guzman M. Impact of hospitalization on patients with nutrition status evaluation at admission Nutr Hosp. 2001;16(1):14–8.

3. Nevett G. Malnutrition of the hospitalised patient—assessment of provision of diet and dietary intake. EDTNA ERCA J. 1997 Oct–Dec;23(4):22–4.

4. de Kruif JT, Vos A. An algorithm for the clinical assessment of nutritional status in hospitalized patients. Br J Nutr. 2003 Oct;90(4):829–36.

5. Sullivan DH, Sun S, Walls RC. Protein-energy undernutrition among elderly hospitalized patients: a prospective study. JAMA. 1999;281(21):2013–9.

6. Elmstahl S, Persson M, Andren M, Blabolil V. Malnutrition in geriatric patients: a neglected problem? J Adv Nurs. 1997 Nov;26(5):851–5.

7. Wendland BE, Greenwood CE, Weinberg I, Young KW. Malnutrition in institutionalized seniors: the iatrogenic component. J Am Geriatr Soc. 2003 Jan;51(1):85–90.

8. Seiler WO. Clinical pictures of malnutrition in ill elderly subjects. Nutrition. 2001 Jun;17(6):496–8.

9. Kelly IE, Tessier S, Cahill A, Morris SE, Crumley A, McLaughlin D, McKee RF, Lean ME. Still hungry in hospital: identifying malnutrition in acute hospital admissions. QJM. 2000;93(2):93–8.

10. Hess CT. Nutritional needs: essential ingredients. How dietary deficiencies can delay wound healing. Nursing. 1995 Apr;25(4):32N.

11. Thomas DR. Specific nutritional factors in wound healing. Adv Wound Care. 1997 Jul–Aug;10(4):40–3; Flanigan KH. Nutritional aspects of wound healing. Adv Wound Care. 1997 May–Jun;10(3):48–52.

12. Avenell A, Handoll HH. A systematic review of protein and energy supplementation for hip fracture aftercare in older people. Eur J Clin Nutr. 2003 Aug;57(8):895–903.

13. Breslow RA, Hallfrisch J, Guy DG, Crawley B, Goldberg AP. The importance of dietary protein in healing pressure ulcers. J Am Geriatr Soc. 1993 Apr;41(4):357–62.

14. Breslow RA, Bergstrom N. Nutritional prediction of pressure ulcers. J Am Diet Assoc. 1994 Nov;94(11):1301–4.

15. Sen CK, Khanna S, Gordillo G, Bagchi D, Bagchi M, Roy S. Oxygen, oxidants, and antioxidants in wound healing: an emerging paradigm Ann. N.Y. Acad. Sci. 2002;957:239–49.

16. Teixeira S. Bioflavonoids: proanthocyanidins and quercetin and their potential roles in treating musculoskeletal conditions. J Orthop Sports Phys Ther. 2002 Jul;32(7):357–63.

17. Khanna S, Venojarvi M, Roy S, Sharma N, Trikha P, Bagchi D, Bagchi M, Sen CK. Dermal wound healing properties of redox-active grape seed proanthocyanidins. Free Radic Biol Med. 2002 Oct 15;33(8):1089–96.

18. Anonymous. Wound care. Vital ingredients. Nurs Times. 1995;91(5):76–8.

19. MacKay D, Miller AL. Nutritional support for wound healing. Altern Med Rev. 2003 Nov;8(4):359–77.

20. Yilmaz C, Erdemli E, Selek H, Kinik H, Arikan M, Erdemli B. The contribution of vitamin C to healing of experimental fractures. Arch Orthop Trauma Surg. 2001 Jul;121(7):426–8.

21. Kubin A, Kaudela K, Jindra R, Alth G, Grunberger W, Wierrani F, Ebermann R. Dehydroascorbic acid in urine as a possible indicator of surgical stress. Ann Nutr Metab. 2003;47(1):1–5.

22. Barnes J, Resch KL, Ernst E. Homeopathy for postoperative ileus? A meta-analysis. J Clin Gastroenterol. 1997;25:628–633; Pinsent RJFH, Baker GPI, Ives G, et al. Does Arnica reduce pain and bleeding after dental extraction? A placebo control led pilot study conducted by the Midland Homoeopathy Research Group (MHRG). Comm Br Hom Res Grp. 1986;15:3–11; Jeffrey SL, Belcher HJ. Use of Arnica to relieve pain after carpal-tunnel release surgery. Altern Ther Health Med. 2002;8:66–68.

23. Long CL, Maull KI, Krishnan RS, Laws HL, Geiger JW, Borghesi L, Franks W, Lawson TC, Sauberlich HE. Ascorbic acid dynamics in the seriously ill and injured. J Surg Res. 2003 Feb;109(2):144–8.

24. Levenson SM, Demetrio AA, Metabolic factors. In: Cohen IK, Diegelmann RF, Linblad WJ, eds. Wound Healing: Biochemical and Clinical Aspects. Philadelphia, PA: WB Saunders Co; 1992:264.

25. Collins N. Adding vitamin C to the wound management mix. Adv Skin Wound Care. 2004 Apr;17(3):109–12.

26. Long CL, Maull KI, Krishnan RS, Laws HL, Geiger JW, Borghesi L, Franks W, Lawson TC, Sauberlich HE. Ascorbic acid dynamics in the seriously ill and injured. J Surg Res. 2003 Feb;109(2):144–8.

27. Gupta A, Singh RL, Raghubir R. Antioxidant status during cutaneous wound healing in immunocompromised rats. Mol Cell Biochem. 2002 Dec;241(1–2):1–7.

28. Baines M, Shenkin A. Use of antioxidants in surgery: a measure to reduce postoperative complications. Curr Opin Clin Nutr Metab Care. 2002;5(6):665–70.

29. Ayello EA, Thomas DR, Litchford MA. Nutritional aspects of wound healing. Home Healthc Nurse. 1999 Nov–Dec;17(11):719–29.

30. Beaulieu AJ, Gohh RY, Han H, Hakas D, Jacques PF, Selhub J, Bostom AG. Enhanced reduction of fasting total homocysteine levels with supraphysiological versus standard multivitamin dose folic acid supplementation in Reahl transplant recipients. Arterioscler Thromb Vasc Biol. 1999 Dec;19(12):2918–21; Badner NH, Freeman D, Spence JD. Preoperative oral B vitamins prevent nitrous oxide-induced postoperative plasma homocysteine increases. Anesth Analg. 2001 Dec;93(6):1507–10.

31. Mazzotta MY. Nutrition and wound healing. J Amer Pod Med Assoc 1994; 84(9):456–62.

32. Andrews M, Gallagher-Allred C. The role of zinc in wound healing. Adv Wound Care. 1999 Apr;12(3):137–8.

33. Faure H, Peyrin JC, Richard MJ, Favier A. Parenteral supplementation with zinc in surgical patients corrects postoperative serum-zinc drop. Biol Trace Elem Res. 1991 Jul;30(1):37–45.

34. Cario E, Jung S, Harder D'Heureuse J, Schulte C, Sturm A, Wiedenmann B, Goebell H, Dignass AU. Effects of exogenous zinc supplementation on intestinal epithelial repair in vitro. Eur J Clin Invest. 2000 May;30(5):419–28.

35. Coster J, McCauley R, Hall J. Role of specific amino acids in nutritional support. ANZ J Surg. 2003 Oct;73(10):846–9.

36. Witte MB, Barbul A. Arginine physiology and its implication for wound healing. Wound Repair Regen. 2003 Nov–Dec;11(6):419–23.

37. Wilmore DW. The effect of glutamine supplementation in patients following elective surgery and accidental injury. J Nutr. 2001 Sep;131(9 Suppl):2543S–9S; Wu G, Meininger CJ, Knabe DA, Bazer FW, Rhoads JM. Arginine nutrition in development, health and disease. Curr Opin Clin Nutr Metab Care. 2000 Jan;3(1):59–66.

38. Brinkhaus B, Lindner M, Schuppan D, Hahn EG. Chemical, pharmacological and clinical profile of the East Asian medical plant Centella asiatica. Phytomedicine. 2000 Oct;7(5):427–48; Suguna L, Sivakumar P, Chandrakasan G. Effects of Centella asiatica extract on dermal wound healing in rats. Indian J Exp Biol. 1996 Dec;34(12):1208–11; Bosse JP, Papillon J, Frenette G, Dansereau J, Cadotte M, Le Lorier J. Clinical study of a new antikeloid agent. Ann Plast Surg. 1979

Jul;3(1):13–21; Maquart FX, Chastang F, Simeon A, Birembaut P, Gillery P, Wegrowski Y. Triterpenes from Centella asiatica stimulate extracellular matrix accumulation in rat experimental wounds. Eur J Dermatol. 1999 Jun;9(4):289–96.

39. Maurer HR. Bromelain: biochemistry, pharmacology and medical use. Cell Mol Life Sci. 2001 Aug;58(9):1234–45.

40. Woolf RM, Snow JW, Walker JH, Broadbent TR. Resolution of an artificially induced hematoma and the influence of a proteolytic enzyme. J Trauma. 1965 Jul;83:491–4; Kamenicek V, Holan P, Franek P. Systemic enzyme therapy in the treatment and prevention of post-traumatic and postoperative swelling. Acta Chir Orthop Traumatol Cech. 2001;68(1):45–9.

41. Petry JJ. Plast Reconstr Surg. 1996; 97(1):233–40; op cit.

42. MacKay D, Miller AL. Altern Med Rev. 2003 Nov;8(4):359–77; op cit; Avijgan M. Phytotherapy: an alternative treatment for non-healing ulcers. J Wound Care. 2004 Apr;13(4):157–8; Gallagher J, Gray M. Is aloe vera effective for healing chronic wounds? J Wound Ostomy Continence Nurs. 2003 Mar;30(2):68–71.

43. Abdullah KM, Abdullah A, Johnson ML, Bilski JJ, Petry K, Redmer DA, Reynolds LP, Grazul-Bilska AT. Effects of Aloe vera on gap junctional intercellular communication and proliferation of human diabetic and nondiabetic skin fibroblasts. J Altern Complement Med. 2003 Oct;9(5):711–8.

44. Chithra P, Sajithlal GB, Chandrakasan G. Influence of Aloe vera on collagen turnover in healing of dermal wounds in rats. Indian J Exp Biol. 1998 Sep;36(9):896–901.

45. Yagi A, Kabash A, Okamura N, Haraguchi H, Moustafa SM, Khalifa TI. Antioxidant, free radical scavenging and anti-inflammatory effects of aloesin derivatives in Aloe vera. Planta Med. 2002 Nov;68(11):957–60.

46. Baumann LS, Spencer J. The effects of topical vitamin E on the cosmetic appearance of scars. Dermatol Surg. 1999 Apr;25(4):311–5.

47. Simon GA, Schmid P, Reifenrath WG, van Ravenswaay T, Stuck BE. Wound healing after laser injury to skin—the effect of occlusion and vitamin E. J Pharm Sci. 1994 Aug;83(8):1101–6; Boissonneault GA, Wang Y, Chung BH. Oxidized low-density lipoproteins delay endothelial wound healing: lack of effect of vitamin E. Ann Nutr Metab. 1995;39(1):1–8.

48. Greenwald DP, Sharzer LA, Padawer J, Levenson SM, Seifter E. Zone II flexor tendon repair: effects of vitamins A, E, beta-carotene. J Surg Res. 1990 Jul;49(1):98–102.

49. Savine R, Sonksen P. Growth hormone—hormone replacement for the somatopause? Horm Res. 2000;53 Suppl 3:37–41.

50. Lee KA, Stotts NA. Support of the growth hormone-somatomedin system to facilitate healing. Heart Lung. 1990;19(2):157–62.

51. Ibid.

52. Everson CA, Crowley WR. Reductions in circulating anabolic hormones induced by sustained sleep deprivation in rats. Am J Physiol Endocrinol Metab. 2004 Jun;286(6):E1060–70.

53. Cauffield JS, Forbes HJ. Dietary supplements used in the treatment of depression, anxiety, and sleep disorders. Lippincotts Prim Care Pract. 1999 May–Jun; 3(3):290–304.

54. Yarrington A, Mehta P. Does sleep promote recovery after bone marrow transplantation? A hypothesis. Pediatr Transplant. 1998 Feb;2(1):51–5.

55. Demling RH, DeSanti L. Involuntary weight loss and the nonhealing wound: the role of anabolic agents. Adv Wound Care. 1999 Jan–Feb;12(1 Suppl):1–14.

56. Savine R, Sonksen P. Growth hormone—hormone replacement for the somatopause? Horm Res. 2000;53 Suppl 3:37–41.

57. Estivariz CF, Ziegler TR. Nutrition and the insulin-like growth factor system. Endocrine. 1997 Aug;7(1):65–71.

58. Manglik S, Cobanov B, Flores G, Nadjafi R, Tayek JA. Serum insulin but not leptin is associated with spontaneous and growth hormone (GH)-releasing hormone-stimulated GH secretion in normal volunteers with and without weight loss. Metabolism. 1998 Sep;47(9):1127–33.

59. Groschl M, Knerr I, Topf HG, Schmid P, Rascher W, Rauh M. Endocrine responses to the oral ingestion of a physiological dose of essential amino acids in humans. J Endocrinol. 2003 Nov;179(2):237–44.

60. Godfrey RJ, Madgwick Z, Whyte GP. The exercise-induced growth hormone response in athletes. Sports Med. 2003;33(8):599–613.

61. Ari Z, Kutlu N, Uyanik BS, Taneli F, Buyukyazi G, Tavli T. Serum testosterone, growth hormone, and insulin-like growth factor-1 levels, mental reaction time, and maximal aerobic exercise in sedentary and long-term physically trained elderly males. Int J Neurosci. 2004 May;114(5):623–37.

62. Xu X, Ingram RL, Sonntag WE. Ethanol suppresses growth hormone-mediated cellular responses in liver slices. Alcohol Clin Exp Res. 1995 Oct;19(5):1246–51; Rojdmark S, Rydvald Y, Aquilonius A, Brismar K. Insulin-like growth factor (IGF)-1 and IGF-binding protein-1 concentrations in serum of normal subjects after alcohol ingestion: evidence for decreased IGF-1 bioavailability. Clin Endocrinol (Oxf). 2000 Mar;52(3):313–8.

63. Everson CA, Crowley WR. Reductions in circulating anabolic hormones induced by sustained sleep deprivation in rats. Am J Physiol Endocrinol Metab. 2004 Jun;286(6):E1060–70; North A. The effect of sleep on wound healing. Ostomy Wound Manage. 1990 Mar–Apr;27:56–8.

❧ Chapter Eight: Holistic Support for Specific Surgical Scenarios

1. Hodges PJ, Kam PC. The peri-operative implications of herbal medicines. Anaesthesia. 2002 Sep;57(9):889–99.

2. Cheng B, Hung CT, Chiu W. Herbal medicine and anaesthesia. Hong Kong Med J. 2002 Apr;8(2):123–30.

3. Lee A, Chui PT, Aun CS, Gin T, Lau AS. Possible interaction between sevoflurane and Aloe vera. Ann Pharmacother. 2004 Oct;38(10):1651–4.

4. Kaye AD, Kucera I, Sabar R. Perioperative anesthesia clinical considerations of alternative medicines. Anesthesiol Clin North America. 2004 Mar;22(1):125–39.

5. Heller AR, Rossel T, Gottschlich B, Tiebel O, Menschikowski M, Litz RJ, Zimmermann T, Koch T. Omega-3 fatty acids improve liver and pancreas function in postoperative cancer patients. Int J Cancer. 2004 Sep 10;111(4):611–6.

6. Sacks GS, Genton L, Kudsk KA. Controversy of immunonutrition for surgical critical-illness patients. Curr Opin Crit Care. 2003 Aug;9(4):300–5.

7. Ornish D. Brown SE. Scherwitz LW. Billings JH. Armstrong WT. Ports TA. McLanahan SM. Kirkeeide RL. Brand RJ. Gould KL. Can lifestyle changes reverse coronary heart disease? The Lifestyle Heart Trial. Lancet. 1990; 336(8708):129–33; Gould KL. Ornish D. Scherwitz L. Brown S. Edens RP. Hess MJ. Mullani N. Bolomey L. Dobbs F. Armstrong WT. et al. Changes in myocardial perfusion abnormalities by positron emission tomography after long-term, intense risk factor modification. JAMA. 1995; 274(11):894–901.

8. Liu S. Stampfer MJ. Manson JE. et al. A prospective study of glycemic load and risk of myocardial infarction in women. FASEB J. 1998;12: A260 (abstr); Jacobs DR. Meyer KA. Kushi LH. Folsom AR. Whole-grain intake may reduce the risk of ischemic heart disease death in postmenopausal women: the Iowa Women's Health Study. Am J Clin Nutr 1998; 68:248–57.

9. Fraser GE. Diet and coronary heart disease; beyond dietary fats and low-density lipoprotein cholesterol. Am J Clin Nutr 1994; 59(suppl): 1117S–23S.

10. Williams A, Riise GC, Anderson BA, Kjellstrom C, Schersten H, Kelly FJ. Compromised antioxidant status and persistent oxidative stress in lung transplant recipients. Free Radic Res. 1999 May;30(5):383–93; Ochoa JJ, Vilchez MJ, Ibanez S, Huertas JR, Palacio MA, Munoz-Hoyos A. Oxidative stress is evident in erythrocytes as well as plasma in patients undergoing heart surgery involving cardiopulmonary bypass. Free Radic Res. 2003 Jan;37(1):11–7.

11. Ochoa JJ, Vilchez MJ, Palacios MA, Garcia JJ, Reiter RJ, Munoz-Hoyos A. Melatonin protects against lipid peroxidation and membrane rigidity in erythrocytes from patients undergoing cardiopulmonary bypass surgery. J Pineal Res. 2003 Sep;35(2):104–8; Nathens AB, Neff MJ, Jurkovich GJ, Klotz P, Farver K, Ruzinski JT, Radella F, Garcia I, Maier RV. Randomized, prospective trial of antioxidant supplementation in critically ill surgical patients. Ann Surg. 2002 Dec;236(6):814–22; Baines M, Shenkin A. Use of antioxidants in surgery: a measure to reduce postoperative complications. Curr Opin Clin Nutr Metab Care. 2002;5(6):665–70.

12. Ochoa JJ, Vilchez MJ, Mataix J, Ibanez-Quiles S, Palacios MA, Munoz-Hoyos A. Oxidative stress in patients undergoing cardiac surgery: comparative study of revascular-

ization and valve replacement procedures. J Surg Res. 2003 May 15;111(2):248–54.

13. Baines M, Shenkin A. Curr Opin Clin Nutr Metab Care. 2002;5(6):665–70; Op cit.

14. Chello M, Mastroroberto P, Romano R, Bevacqua E, Pantaleo D, Ascione R, Marchese AR, Spampinato N. Protection by coenzyme Q10 from myocardial reperfusion injury during coronary artery bypass grafting. Ann Thorac Surg. 1994 Nov; 58(5):1427–32; Chello M, Mastroroberto P, Romano R, Castaldo P, Bevacqua E, Marchese AR. Protection by coenzyme Q10 of tissue reperfusion injury during abdominal aortic cross-clamping. J Cardiovasc Surg (Torino). 1996 Jun;37(3):229–35.

15. Rosenfeldt F, Marasco S, Lyon W, Wowk M, Sheeran F, Bailey M, Esmore D, Davis B, Pick A, Rabinov M, Smith J, Nagley P, Pepe S. Coenzyme Q10 therapy before cardiac surgery improves mitochondrial function and in vitro contractility of myocardial tissue. J Thorac Cardiovasc Surg. 2005 Jan;129(1):25–32; Rosenfeldt F, Miller F, Nagley P, Hadj A, Marasco S, Quick D, Sheeran F, Wowk M, Pepe S. Response of the senescent heart to stress: clinical therapeutic strategies and quest for mitochondrial predictors of biological age. Ann N Y Acad Sci. 2004 Jun;1019:78–84; Rosenfeldt FL, Pepe S, Linnane A, Nagley P, Rowland M, Ou R, Marasco S, Lyon W. The effects of ageing on the response to cardiac surgery: protective strategies for the ageing myocardium. Biogerontology. 2002;3(1–2):37–40.

16. Priebe D, McDiarmid T, Mackler L, Tudiver F. Do glucosamine or chondroitin cause regeneration of cartilage in osteoarthritis? J Fam Pract. 2003 Mar;52(3):237–9.

17. Hungerford DS, Jones LC. Glucosamine and chondroitin sulfate are effective in the management of osteoarthritis. J Arthroplasty. 2003 Apr;18(3 Suppl 1):5–9; Creamer P. Osteoarthritis pain and its treatment. Curr Opin Rheumatol. 2000 Sep;12(5):450–5.

18. Pribitkin ED, Boger G. Herbal therapy: what every facial plastic surgeon must know. Arch Facial Plast Surg. 2001 Apr–Jun;3(2):127–32.

19. TerKonda RP. Incorporating skin care into a facial plastic surgery practice. Facial Plast Surg. 2004 Feb;20(1):3–9.

20. Hofer SO, Molema G, Hermens RA, Wanebo HJ, Reichner JS, Hoekstra HJ. The effect of surgical wounding on tumour development. Eur J Surg Oncol 1999; 25(3):231–43; Gutman M, Singh RK, Price JE, Fan D, Fidler IJ. Accelerated growth of human colon cancer cells in nude mice undergoing liver regeneration. Invasion & Metastasis. 14(1–6):362–71, 1994–95.

21. Calder PC. Long-chain n-3 fatty acids and inflammation: potential application in surgical and trauma patients. Braz J Med Biol Res. 2003 Apr;36(4):433–46.

22. Hardman WE. Omega-3 fatty acids to augment cancer therapy. J Nutr. 2002 Nov;132(11 Suppl):3508S–3512S.

23. McMurry JF Jr. Wound healing with diabetes mellitus. Better glucose control for better wound healing in diabetes. Surg Clin North Am. 1984 Aug;64(4):769–78; Collins N. Diabetes, nutrition, and wound healing. Adv Skin Wound Care. 2003 Nov;16(6):291–4.

24. UKPDS group. Effect of intensive blood-glucose control with sulphonylureas or insulin compared with conventional treatment and risks of complications in patients

with type 2 diabetes. Lancet. 1998 Sep 12;352(9131):837–53; Mousley M. Diabetes and its effect on wound healing and patient care. Nurs Times. 2003 Oct 21–27;99(42):70, 73–4; Wallace LK, Starr NJ, Leventhal MJ, Estafanous FG. Hyperglycaemia on ICU admission after CABG is associated with increased risk of mediastinitis or wound infection. Anesthesiology 1996;85 (Suppl):A286.

25. Terranova A. The effects of diabetes mellitus on wound healing. Plast Surg Nurs. 1991 Spring;11(1):20–5.
26. Thorell A, Nygren J, Ljungqvist O. Insulin resistance: a marker of surgical stress. Curr Opin Clin Nutr Metab Care. 1999 Jan;2(1):69–78.
27. Cefalu WT, Hu FB. Role of chromium in human health and in diabetes. Diabetes Care. 2004 Nov;27(11):2741–51.
28. Hipkiss AR. Carnosine, a protective, anti-ageing peptide? Int J Biochem Cell Biol. 1998 Aug;30(8):863–8.
29. Simopoulos AP. Essential fatty acids in health and chronic disease. American Journal of Clinical Nutrition. 1999;70(3 Suppl):560S-569S; Simopoulos AP. Evolutionary aspects of omega-3 fatty acids in the food supply. Prostaglandins Leukotrienes & Essential Fatty Acids. 1999; 60(5–6):421–9.
30. Ito Y, Shimizu H, Yoshimura T, Ross RK, et al. Serum concentrations of carotenoids, alpha-tocopherol, fatty acids, and lipid peroxides among Japanese in Japan, and Japanese and Caucasians in the US. International Journal for Vitamin & Nutrition Research. 1999; 69(6):385–95; Kelly FJ. The metabolic role of n-3 polyunsaturated fatty acids: relationship to human disease. Comparative Biochemistry & Physiology A—Comparative Physiology. 1991; 98(3–4):581–5; Simopoulos AP. Robinson J. The Omega Plan. New York: HarperCollins, 1998: p. 29.
31. Stoof TJ, Korstanje MJ, Bilo HJ, Starink TM, Hulsmans RF, Donker AJ. Does fish oil protect Reahl function in cyclosporin-treated psoriasis patients? J Intern Med. 1989 Dec;226(6):437–41.

Chapter Nine: Life after the Knife

1. Seamen DR. The diet-induced proinflammatory state: a cause of chronic pain and other degenerative diseases? J Manipulative Physiol Ther. 2002 Mar–Apr;25(3): 168–79.

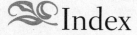# Index